# What You Should Know About Medical Lab Tests

# What You Should Know About Medical Lab Tests

Bernard Kliman, M.D.
and Raymond Vermette, M.S.,
with Ernest Kolowrat

Thomas Y. Crowell, Publishers
Established 1834 New York

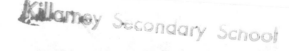

FIRST EDITION

LIBRARY OF CONGRESS CATALOGING IN PUBLICATION DATA

Kliman, Bernard
  What you should know about medical lab tests.

  Includes index.
  1. Diagnosis, Laboratory. I. Vermette, Raymond, joint author. II. Kolowrat, Ernest, joint author. III. Title. [DNLM: 1. Diagnosis, Laboratory—Popular works. QY4.3 K65w]
  RB37.K57      616.07'5      79–7092
  ISBN 0–690–01831–2

79 80 81 82 83 10 9 8 7 6 5 4 3 2 1

# Contents

# Acknowledgments

This book represents the combined efforts of many individuals for whose invaluable assistance we are deeply grateful. Our special thanks to Oliver Swan, our agent; to Hugh Rawson, our editor; to F. Thomas Kolowrat for suggesting the need for this book; to Gerald J. Phaneuf, M.D., pathologist, for his review of the manuscript and countless recommendations for clarifying the correlations between laboratory testing and various disease conditions; to Richard W. Kocon, Ph.D., for providing many useful ideas and suggesting valuable reference sources; to Sue Atkins and Janet Bouret for successfully deciphering our illegible scrawls in typing the manuscript; and to our respective families, whose patience, understanding, and encouragement enabled us to take on this project and see it through to completion.

Bernard Kliman, M.D.
Raymond Vermette, M.S., M.B.A.
Ernest Kolowrat

# For Your Quick Reference

Editor's Note: There is no single, standard way in which all medical laboratories group their test results. How your results will be grouped may depend on what tests your doctor orders and on the technology and equipment used by the testing laboratory. The tests in this book have been grouped primarily by their common relevance to the same organ or to similar bodily functions. This grouping provides for a logical, step-by-step presentation of the complex workings of the body. Many laboratories also use similar groupings.

# 1
# Why This Book Now?

Ten years ago, most of the people who walked into my office rarely asked probing questions. What they basically wanted to know was, were they healthy? Those who were not wanted me to tell them how to get well again—what pills to take, what further examinations to undergo, what surgery might be needed, and whatever else it might take to restore their health.

I was the doctor. Despite my relative youth, I knew best. It was up to me to make them well. The most they could do was to follow what the doctor ordered.

Today, not all patients are quite so unquestioning, despite my additional years of experience. I am seeing more and more individuals who want to participate actively in getting well, or in just staying well. They have been exposed to a number of medically oriented self-help or self-improvement books. They have heard about the virtues of getting a second opinion. They might even have a very definite opinion of their own. They want to know everything possible about their case. No detail is too small or too technical. Even if they do not quite understand what I am saying, they want to be in a position of being able to make up their own minds about the condition of their health.

Medical testing is one area where I am getting more and more questions. Some of my patients have received insurance statements showing charges for tests with such strange-sounding names as chem-profile, total $T_4$ and CBC. Since they indirectly had to pay for them, they feel they have a right to know about them.

Some of my patients may have even glimpsed a computerized sheet on my desk of their own chem-profile, with a list of perhaps twenty-one different test names and numerical values. The names and numbers probably did not mean very much to them. But this has rarely kept them from showing a healthy curiosity, especially about those tests visibly marked as abnormal.

I welcome this development, this desire on the part of patients to know everything possible about their condition, and to participate actively in their treatment. The process of getting well or staying well is a very intricate one. The doctor cannot and should not be expected to do it alone. It has to be a partnership in which both doctor and patient do their share.

As a doctor, I have medical expertise and experience acquired over many years of highly specialized training. My patients, on the other hand, have an equally important expertise: knowing themselves, as only they can. By telling me about themselves—how they feel, what hurts them, what makes them feel better—I can best make my diagnosis and recommendations for treatment. They, in turn, are likely to be more responsive as patients if I explain to them, in the greatest detail possible, the reasons for my diagnosis and treatment.

## Doctor–Patient Relationship

For a true partnership to exist between doctor and patient, there has to be a free flow of information in both directions. And here is where we often hit a snag. While there is practically no barrier to keep your doctor from understanding you as a patient, you might be at a disadvantage in trying to understand your doctor. Sooner or later, the doctor's explanations will involve medical language and concepts with which few patients are familiar.

This is especially true in the area of medical testing. It is a highly specialized field. Most patients may have heard of tests for cholesterol, glucose, or triglycerides, even if they are not sure exactly what they mean. But how much do they know about bilirubin, alkaline phosphatase, or hematocrit? These could turn out to be far more important in their individual cases than any of the more familiar tests.

There are more than fifty common laboratory tests which could play a decisive role in any diagnosis and treatment. Over five hundred other tests are done far less frequently, but nevertheless could prove important in individual cases.

Most doctors do not have the time to explain very much about your tests. An explanation could well take longer than the entire examination.

With a waiting room full of patients, doctors often are in no position to attempt to teach a quick course in biology. A broad generalization is usually the best you can expect.

For example: "Your urine and blood chemistry are fine. Only your red blood cells are slightly on the low side, but you should not worry about it." Or: "Your creatinine—that is, your kidney-function test—was a bit high. I would like to run it again."

Why in the world should you *not* worry if your red blood cells were low? Why does the doctor want to run the creatinine test again? It can all be so frustrating.

There are also doctors who believe that your test results are not your concern. A little knowledge, they warn, could be a dangerous thing; you might draw the wrong conclusions and worry needlessly. After all, it has taken them years of training and experience to interpret test results properly. So, they tell you nothing.

And they have a valid point. Unless you do get a *complete* explanation, you might be better off not knowing anything at all. Even if they did have the time, most doctors probably could not give you such a thorough explanation. They are usually familiar with these tests in terms of highly technical language, and would find it difficult to translate them into everyday words and concepts.

Other than the doctor, there really is hardly anyplace you can now go to find out about laboratory testing. Except for the highly technical texts, there is little that is complete on the subject in encyclopedias, biology books, and other medical writing aimed at the general public. Moreover, some of the information on medical testing is so recent that even the technical reference works are not always up to date. Almost every day there seem to be new discoveries and advances in laboratory testing, making it one of the fastest-developing fields in medicine.

## The Testing Revolution

It was not too many years ago that a doctor might have given you a complete annual physical without ordering a single lab test on your blood. A urinalysis might have been done as part of the routine, but any additional tests would have been ordered very sparingly—probably only when the doctor suspected a serious illness. Even then, the number of tests ordered would have been small, perhaps only two or three. Under no circumstances would the doctor have ordered the extensive batteries of tests that are almost routine today.

The fact that some of these tests had not been developed twenty-five or even ten years ago is only part of the reason. Perhaps the main reason was expense. A whole battery of tests would have been prohibitively expensive for most patients.

In those days, tests were carried out in a relatively tedious way that is familiar to anyone who has taken high school chemistry—at a stand-up desk, with test tubes, pipettes, Bunsen burners, and similar equipment. Done individually and by hand, each test might have cost the patient five dollars. And that was back in pre-inflation times.

Today, for about twenty-five to thirty-five dollars, you can get perhaps as many as forty such tests done as standard part of your physical examination and laboratory evaluation. Obviously, medical testing, along with the after-hours long-distance phone call, is one of the few bargains still around!

The reason for the bargain? Highly advanced technology. Many of the key tests today are done automatically, often on futuristic-looking machines once seen only in science-fiction movies. Although technicians are always there supervising, often the only time they need actually handle a specimen is when they remove a portion for analysis.

By far the bulk of all medical testing is ordered directly by doctors. Yet, with such ready availability of low-cost laboratory testing that can effectively screen your health, other avenues for bringing these tests to the public have opened up.

In California, for instance, many people are availing themselves of special mini-physicals, usually offered at their place of work. The physicals are administered by a nurse and consist of selected groups of blood and urine tests, plus blood pressure, chest X-ray, and an electrocardiogram. The computer printout of the results, which goes directly to the individual, does not attempt to diagnose; rather, it points out any abnormalities which should be looked into by a physician.

In Florida, you can actually walk into certain health-food stores where a uniformed nurse will take blood and urine samples, count your pulse, and measure your blood pressure. You can expect to pay about twenty-five dollars, and by the next day you'll receive a computer printout of the results.

Of course, it is up to you to figure out what it all means. This could prove to be a very risky business. Even most physicians would hesitate to make a definitive diagnosis on the basis of lab tests alone. If some of your test results are not normal, you may go through a lot of needless worry. Needless because, as you will see in the next chapter, so-called abnormal results do not necessarily mean that there is something wrong with you. On the other hand, just because all your results are normal does not mean you have an ironclad guarantee of being healthy. You may, in fact, need to see a physician more than does the person with some of those test abnormalities. It takes a lot of training and judgment to recognize exactly what is important among laboratory test results.

## The Importance of Testing

Of all the hundreds of different laboratory tests your doctor can choose from, the most common are the basic screens. These consist of a urinalysis, with a half-dozen different tests; a blood chemistry profile, which includes up to twenty-one different tests; and a complete blood count, which usually adds up to another dozen tests. Two important points to keep in mind:

First, urine and blood tests are not merely checks to see whether your urine and blood are all right. They are much more than that. Your blood and your urine accumulate from throughout your body. In one way or another, they have come in contact with virtually every cell of your body, and thus carry within them many of the countless by-products of the various organs. By examining your blood and urine for different factors, your doctor is, in effect, taking a look at some of the most inaccessible organs of your body.

Second, your doctor will rarely, if ever, order just these screening tests without giving you a thorough physical before making a diagnosis. During the physical, the doctor has more tangible ways of checking your organs and the state of your health in general. These are all probably familiar to you. They range from looking into your eyes, ears, and throat to listening to your heart, feeling for your liver—and, always, asking a lot of questions.

Thus, you are really getting two physicals: the blood and urine screening tests and the doctor's actual examination. What usually happens is that one confirms or amplifies the findings of the other.

For example, if I give you an examination and find you in top-notch health, the chances are that your tests will come back essentially normal, confirming those findings. If, on the other hand, you enter my office with a yellowish tinge to your skin and eyeballs, and complaining of nausea and pain in the abdominal area, the blood and urine tests would most likely confirm my impression of jaundice due to liver disorder. I would probably order several more specific liver-function tests to pinpoint the exact nature of the problem.

Most cases, of course, are not so clear-cut. Sometimes, a suspicion is confirmed by the lab tests. At other times, a suspicion can be laid to rest by those same tests.

Purely from the doctor's point of view, lab tests have still another purpose. By providing a measurable record of a patient's state of health at a particular time, they protect the doctor from unwarranted malpractice suits. They also make it more likely that a second opinion is going to be pretty much the same as the first.

But protecting the doctor by confirming a diagnosis is by no means the main reason for such a large assortment of tests: the best doctors are more intent on helping patients than constantly worrying about being sued. The main reason for these tests, most doctors would probably agree, is that they may actually uncover illnesses in patients which would otherwise go undetected—perhaps until it was too late. Many diseases, such as leukemia or diabetes, sometimes make themselves known through subtle changes in the blood or urine months or even years before they could be detected through a routine physical examination.

Some illnesses could be life-threatening, or could be merely something to watch. Early diagnosis through medical tests may enable the doctor to head off the disease altogether—or to start treatment at a stage when the patient will have an incomparably better chance for recovery.

Of course, the basic screening tests also indicate to the doctor what additional tests should be ordered. By looking at a test result that appears to be abnormal, the doctor is in a position to move closer to the source of the problem. Here, the doctor has all those other hundreds of tests to choose from, some of which may be essential for making a precise diagnosis. These further tests could even spare the patient exploratory surgery or other inconvenient or costly medical procedures.

Once the diagnosis has been made, specific blood and urine tests are often used to monitor how well the patient is recovering. Many of the same tests which uncovered the disease can tell the doctor how effective the treatment is. Other tests can help find the best levels of medication, which at times can also be a life-and-death question.

Sometimes, laboratory testing can even prevent a disease. Those who are exposed to poisonous chemicals and fumes while at work are being increasingly protected by periodic testing of their blood and urine. By detecting and measuring any toxic substances in the body, appropriate steps can be taken before dangerous levels are reached.

Similar tests can be used to discover substance abuse, such as whether a youngster has been sniffing airplane glue, which can be every bit as lethal as the most dangerous industrial poisons. In cases of drug overdoses, there are tests to find out what kind of substance a person in a coma has taken, so that the right antidote can be administered.

There seem to be no limits to how far medical testing can advance. There are already several promising tests to detect various forms of cancer through a simple blood sample, far earlier than through other means. There are experimental ultra-thin computerized probes that can be inserted in an artery of the arm to continuously monitor the delicate balance of several key chemicals in the blood. There was a time when a whole laboratory of technicians could not have managed such a task.

The day may come, in the next century, when you will be able to stand in front of a machine which, without drawing a drop of blood, will be able to perform hundreds of crucial tests. Within seconds, you will get a printout of your health, revealing your condition with a degree of accuracy and wealth of detail beyond anything possible in a present-day examination.

## Too Much Testing?

Despite the obvious benefits to the patient from the "testing revolution," there are critics who claim that there is too much testing; that many of the tests are inappropriate and add a needless financial burden to the costs of medical care.

In virtually any field which grows as fast as laboratory testing has in the past several years, there are bound to be problems. Some doctors may indeed order tests that are not needed or are inappropriate to the apparent physical condition of the patient while perhaps overlooking other tests that could prove useful.

Such questionable testing, however, is not usually motivated by a desire for personal gain by unscrupulous individuals. For any physician, it is a tremendous challenge to keep up to date with what is happening in medical laboratory testing—the new tests, the new concepts, the new applications. No wonder that some physicians may order too many tests simply because they want to minimize the possibility of overlooking tests that could prove crucial to a correct diagnosis. Like detectives, some physicians are more adept than others in following up on the right clues and solving the more difficult cases.

Another point to keep in mind: it may actually be cheaper for you as a patient to have a complete screen of blood and urine tests—perhaps as many as twenty—than the four or five your physician may actually consider as vital. The testing technology is such that it is easier to do an entire battery of screening tests on automated equipment than to manually process fewer individual tests. And the bulk of medical laboratory testing today does consist of these automated screening tests, at a lower unit cost per test than non-automated tests.

## Why *You* Should Know

Whatever the future may hold for medical testing, there are compelling reasons why you should know about the tests available to you now. These are your own tests, a part of you, reflecting on what is happening in your body. By knowing more about them, you can understand better what your doctor is trying to do for you—and become a better patient.

The results of your various tests are like a report card. Even the format is similar. Instead of subjects, there are the names of the tests. Instead of grades, there are numerical values relative to normal levels. Instead of a range from failing to superior, there is a range from the lower limit to the upper limit. And, as on a report card, all the failing grades —or values outside the normal ranges—are clearly indicated, with an asterisk or other eye-catching device.

The purpose of a report card is to show you not only how you are doing but also where you can improve. So too, we need some measurable benchmark to evaluate our health, and in this case our report card is a medical test printout.

True, some of the values on your medical test printout can be improved only through medication or other intervention by your doctor. Still, it is good to know how you are doing and to gain confidence in the process. As you see yourself making progress in measurable terms, reflected in subsequent lab results, such as a declining uric acid level if you have a case of gout, you will feel rewarded for following the doctor's advice. You might even be prompted to still greater cooperation, especially if the treatment is less than pleasant.

Of course, not everybody improves. In that case, you might want to be the first to know. And if you do not want to know, you can be sure that your doctor is not likely to insist. The right to know does not mean giving up the right not to know.

Most of the time, you yourself will be able to do something to improve your laboratory report card. None of your test results need even be abnormal. Maybe your cholesterol and triglycerides are creeping up to the upper range of normal. In that case, it is just as important that your doctor tell you this as it is for you to know when you are a few pounds overweight. Weight, cholesterol, and triglycerides—as well as a number of other elevated test values—usually can be considerably improved through exercise, diet, and other changes in your lifestyle.

This all takes a lot of effort. Knowing what these test values really mean for your health may convince you dramatically that such an effort is well worth it. And subsequent test printouts can give you additional motivation to continue.

The more you know about medical testing, the better off you may be in general. You may learn how to avoid some of the hazards of our technological environment which can so drastically alter your test results —and, in fact, cause severe illness. You may learn how to give your doctor highly pertinent information which you might otherwise have thought unimportant, even under direct prodding. Such information could provide your doctor with the missing link that makes a proper diagnosis possible.

There is still another reason for knowing as much about medical testing as you possibly can. It will give you a unique view of how your body works; what principles it seems to obey; how intricate are its countless processes; how delicate the balance between functioning and malfunctioning. You will recognize how precious your health is and begin to care for it properly and with the devotion it deserves.

# 2
# Am I Normal?

We live at a time when it is stylish to be different. To be normal or average is a bore. Many people take pride in flaunting their individuality —whether it is the result of ethnic or racial heritage, or just a matter of personal taste and quirks.

You would be surprised how quickly this desire to be anything but average or normal evaporates the instant most people walk into my office. Almost desperately, what the patient wants to know more than anything else is: Am I normal? Is my blood pressure normal? How about my blood and urine tests? How about my health in general? Yes, in a doctor's office, almost everybody aspires to be normal. There are relatively few exceptions—people who would have nothing but contempt at being declared normal. Physically, the exceptions usually are highly trained individuals who lead disciplined lives and enjoy superb health. They believe that in our industrialized, sedentary society to be normal means to be at least partly sick.

To what extent they may be right remains for future research to decide. In at least one respect, they do have a valid point. Whether or not you are normal depends on how your results compare to those of other people from the area where you live who are considered to be healthy. In fact, the standard of comparison may often be derived from among the employees at the laboratory where your tests are being performed.

The main purpose of this chapter is to put you at ease; to keep you from worrying even if your tests do not at first glance appear to be normal. You are first and foremost an individual, with your own idiosyncrasies. This will be reflected in laboratory tests as in any other aspect of life. You do not have to measure up in every respect to qualify as "normal."

Here is a simple example: It is November in Massachusetts and it is cold. Everybody is wearing a topcoat, yet you are walking around in just a jacket. People think you are weird and give you curious looks. To them, you seem anything but normal. What they do not know is that you spent the past two years in Greenland with the Air Force and this weather feels just fine to you. Even if you had not spent that time in snowy Greenland, your tolerance for cold weather need not necessarily mean that there is something wrong with you. It could be just the way you are.

With somebody else, this sort of behavior could be a sign of an overactive thyroid gland, an excess of growth hormone, or even a fever, and a doctor might well find the situation in need of further checking.

You should remember that not all the healthy people sampled are entered into the calculation when averaging out what is normal. Just as with that fellow who happened to be feeling warm in the November cold, we know that there are always small numbers of healthy individuals whose norms will be considerably out of range of almost everybody else's. Their values are "normal" only for them. These people are not included in the normal sample against which you will be measured. Statistically, the 5 percent—or one out of every twenty—who fall on either the high end or the low end of the sample tested are removed from consideration when the so-called normal range is calculated.

That means you have a one-in-twenty chance of having an abnormal result and still being normal. But here is another consideration. Let us say that a detailed survey of some forty blood and urine tests is performed. Just from the statistical point of view, you could have two test results outside the normal range and still be normal. Thus, the likelihood is that at least some of your tests may turn out abnormal regardless of how normal you really are. In fact, even if you are perfectly healthy, the chances that *all* your screening tests will be normal are only about one in three.

Not accurate enough? What is remarkable is that the system works as well as it does. The sample on which the normal range is based usually consists of between 100 and 200 people. When you consider that these people serve as a reference point for more than 200 million people, you begin to appreciate the magic of statistics!

## How Do You Measure Up?

It is understandable why laboratory testing holds a certain mystery for most people. Once your sample has been collected, it is rushed off to some anonymous laboratory where it is put through paces most people could not even begin to imagine. What comes back often is a report full of seemingly undecipherable names alongside equally incomprehensible measurements.

Of these measurements, perhaps the least familiar are milliEquivalents and units. MilliEquivalents are used to measure such minerals in your body as sodium, potassium, and chloride. A milliEquivalent is a measure not only of quantity, but also of the ability of the mineral to interact with other materials of equivalent but opposite electrical charges in the body. Units are a measure of the capacity of some of your body's regulator substances, or enzymes, such as SGOT, SGPT, LDH (about which more later) to generate specific chemical products. These units are based on the same idea of general activity as the units you may have seen on a penicillin prescription. Whether units or milliEquivalents, it is more important for you to know where your test results fall in respect to the normal ranges than what precisely these technical terms do mean.

The rest of the measurements are relatively straightforward, utilizing the metric system. Most of the blood constituents are measured in milligrams per 100 milliliters or per deciliter. A deciliter is one-tenth of a liter, or 100 milliliters. Although many laboratories are beginning to use the deciliter designation in reporting test results, we have retained the more familiar 100 milliliter format. In either case, they amount to the same thing.

Now, these are very small quantities. A hundred milliliters is a little less than a quarter of a pint. A milligram, on the other hand, is one-millionth of a kilogram, or one-thousandth of a gram. That is about the weight of a thin hair less than an inch long. Sometimes, even this proves to be too large a unit. There are further subdivisions into micrograms, nanograms, and picograms. Respectively, they are one-millionth, one-billionth, and one-trillionth of a gram. Which is really splitting hairs!

You might notice that some of the normal ranges indicated on your printout vary somewhat from the ranges indicated in this book. This does not mean that either the book or the lab is mistaken. The two sets of ranges merely reflect the somewhat different circumstances under which the tests are performed in different laboratories.

For example: A laboratory that does most of its work by mail—with perhaps a two-day delay in receiving the specimen—will get somewhat different results than a local lab that has all the samples delivered over a relatively short distance on practically an hourly basis. The equipment in the respective laboratories may also be slightly different, and the population on which the reference standards are based may also have some unique characteristics.

But such variations will be relatively slight. The range that is correct for your purposes is the one indicated on the test report from your laboratory.

If your result is slightly or even far off, it could also be because of a mistake. Most of the mistakes happen before the specimen reaches the laboratory. They are usually caused by improper handling or inadequate preservation of the specimen. Perhaps it has been let stand too long, or exposed to undue heat. Perhaps the technician did not draw the sample properly in the first place.

And laboratories do make mistakes. In performing thousands of tests daily, the possibility that something, somewhere, will go slightly wrong cannot be ruled out. Reputable laboratories go to great lengths to ensure accuracy of their work. The autoanalyzer, which can complete each hour a battery of twenty-one tests on a hundred different samples, is constantly being checked. Approximately every ten minutes a test sample with known values is passed through to check its accuracy. And about every fifteen to twenty minutes other reference samples are run through to check the machine's calibration.

If your doctor suspects that an abnormal test result is due to a technical error, the test will be repeated. It will not cost you anything, and the chances of a random error twice in a row are remote.

## Your Tests Are What You Are

You do not have to be unhealthy to sometimes have various abnormal readings. There are a number of factors besides disease which may be affecting your body and shifting your results into the abnormal range. Disease just happens to be by far the most prominent of all factors that affect your test results.

What are some of the other factors? There are many, but perhaps the most prominent include undue physical exercise or exertion; emotional stress or pressure; exposure to excessive cold or heat; menstruation or pregnancy. All are basically activities or conditions which may not be entirely normal for you. It should then not be surprising that these variables can result in abnormal test results.

For instance, if you have just finished strenuous exercise your urine sample may contain excessive protein, ketones, and even myoglobin. As you will see in the chapter on urine, each of these substances could be a sign of severe illness. Yet, after exercise, you might have all three in your urine and still be a picture of health.

The effects of menstruation are well known. Because of the periodic blood loss, women often have low iron levels in their blood. Doctors usually consider this normal and prescribe an iron supplement. If, on the other hand, a woman past menopause—or a man—happens to have low blood iron, it could be serious. The doctor will want to check further for the possibility of intestinal bleeding or some other form of hemorrhaging.

What you eat also can affect your laboratory test results. This is the reason for fasting for several hours before blood and urine specimens are taken. Your doctor wants to make sure that some of the tests will not just be measuring what you had for your last meal.

For example, coffee may cause a false positive test for bilirubin in your urine. The sugar level in your blood, taken an hour after eating, could appear to be in the diabetic range if judged by a fasting standard. Your triglycerides may show up abnormally high even several hours after eating. It takes triglycerides about twelve to fifteen hours to clear out of the bloodstream. As for some of the longer-range effects of diet, your blood urea nitrogen (BUN) can be substantially elevated as a result of a high-protein diet heavy in meats. Although BUN elevations usually are a sign of serious kidney disease, in this case your doctor would probably tell you not to worry—if you told him or her your dietary habits.

Even more dramatic effects on your test results may be caused by medication. This is one reason why the doctor will always ask whether you are taking any medication. Unfortunately, many people do not think of birth control pills or aspirin as medication. Yet both can make a number of key test results appear abnormal.

For instance, birth control pills can sometimes increase levels of the enzyme SGOT and thereby give a false warning that something might be wrong with your heart or liver. Aspirin may have a marked effect on how long it takes your blood to clot. Antibiotics, laxatives, and other, less-well-known drugs also can throw some of your test results into the abnormal range.

Age can have a telling effect on your test results. As people get older, their test values gradually tend to depart from the accepted norms. This seems to be a part of the normal aging process and should be no cause for special concern. However, all such changes are not inevitable. Many elderly people who are committed to healthy lifestyles may have better test values than they did in their overindulgent youth!

In at least one respect, the aging process brings improvement for more than half of our population. In most women, iron levels come up to normal after menopause—and stay normal.

This all goes to show that we are always changing. However, our tests only show us at one particular point in time. The changes they reflect do not necessarily indicate disease, but the fluctuations we undergo from day to day, even from moment to moment.

Thus, our test results quickly become obsolete. About the only use your doctor will have for your present results a year from now will be as a point of reference, as a basis of comparison for whatever your test results may be then.

## High End or Low?

When your test results come back to your doctor from the laboratory, any abnormal values are usually marked by an asterisk or similar eye-catching device. The purpose of the asterisk is not to alarm the patient but to alert the doctor.

Often, the opposite turns out to be the case. The patient gets a glimpse of all those asterisks and becomes upset. The doctor might merely glance at them and dismiss them in short order.

Negligence? ignorance? lack of interest? you may ask. Most likely not. What your doctor is probably looking for are not any abnormalities, but those changes that are truly significant.

And how does the doctor make such judgments? There is no hard-and-fast rule that applies to evaluating all the various blood and urine tests. The only way your doctor can tell whether you are dangerously abnormal is through experience and training. A complete physical examination is essential as a reference point against which the various test values can be judged.

Here is a case in point: Sodium and potassium are two vital salts in your body. Without them, life could not continue. Yet you can have relatively lower levels of sodium in your blood, with no ill effects, than of potassium. The reason? Most of your potassium is stored in body tissues, with comparatively little of it actually in your bloodstream. If you register an *abnormally* low amount of potassium in your blood, that means that your body stores of this vital mineral already have been greatly depleted. And that could prove dangerous. With sodium, most of it is in the bloodstream in the first place. Below-normal sodium values may not signify any serious drain of sodium from your body tissues.

The danger of low potassium levels in your body points up the fact that low levels on your tests can often be just as dangerous as the highs. This is true even of such constituents as cholesterol and glucose, where the dire warnings are almost exclusively against high levels.

Take cholesterol. Too much supposedly leads to heart attacks. But too little can be a sign of severe liver disorders as well as of other serious diseases. Sugar, or glucose, is another case in point. Too much of it in your blood is a sign of diabetes. Yet too little can signify hypoglycemia —a disorder that can be every bit as disabling as diabetes.

You will see on your printout that the range between high and low in some laboratory tests is very narrow. The range for calcium is 8.5 to 10.5 milligrams per 100 milliliters. A mere 20 percent separates the high and the low end of the scale. Yet, to be either slightly high or slightly low can mean severe health problems, possibly ranging from glandular disorders on the high side to kidney disorders and bone disease on the low side.

Triglycerides offer a dramatic contrast. There is no special danger attached to being slightly on the high side or slightly on the low side. The normal range is from 50 to 170 milligrams per 100 milliliters. Three hundred percent separates the upper and lower limits. That means one person can have more than three times as high a triglyceride level as another, and both will still fall within normal limits.

With such a wide gap between the upper and lower end of normal on so many tests, where should yours fall? What are *your* optimal values?

Again, nobody is in a position to tell you exactly. Let us take cholesterol, simply because it is probably the best known of our blood constituents. The typical range is 140 to 265 milligrams per 100 milliliters. We know that, all other factors being equal, the lower your cholesterol the better your chances of avoiding heart disease.

The key is, *all other factors being equal.* Such is rarely the situation. For example, we know that the Bantu in Africa have, for some unknown reason, enviably low cholesterol levels. Yet, because all other factors are not equal, their life span is about twenty years less than ours.

Yes, you should try to have as low a cholesterol level as possible— consistent with an acceptable lifestyle. There is little point in imposing severe deprivation on yourself just to reduce your cholesterol from 200 to 150. You may be one of those people for whom a higher cholesterol level is perfectly natural, with no serious, long-term consequences. All things considered, you may in fact be better off with the higher figure, since stress, which plays a role in heart disease, may be compounded by severe diets and other restrictions.

Your own tests from previous years may be an excellent guide for detecting any potential problems—especially tests that have broad normal ranges, such as cholesterol and triglycerides. What your physician is looking for, in any overall examination, are signs of significant changes from the last time you were examined.

For example, if you gained 20 pounds in the past year, the physician would want to know why. Are you exercising less? Eating more? Have you given up smoking? Any other lifestyle changes? If you are a woman, are you pregnant? Or, is this weight gain an indication of a potential disease state, such as retention of water by your body's cells?

By the same token, if your triglycerides have been a steady 80 milligrams per 100 milliliters in previous years, the physician might raise questions if they suddenly show up as 150 this year—even though that is still well within the normal range. Did you fast long enough before your blood sample was drawn? Has your lifestyle changed? Are you taking any medication which could be responsible for the sudden jump? Or, is this sudden jump an early warning of some disease—even though you are still within the range of normal?

On the other hand, perhaps even a higher triglyceride reading of 160 would be unlikely to arouse your physician's concern if tests in previous years had consistently resulted in similar readings. Again: What is normal for one person may be abnormal for someone else.

Above all, you should not become unduly concerned about your test results. You have seen not only how helpful they can be, but also what their limitations are. Make the most of knowing about them and understanding them.

# 3
# Your Most Basic Tests

Height, weight, and temperature. These are household words, familiar to everyone. Have you ever thought of them as tests? As indicators of your health, they have a great deal in common with laboratory testing. In any routine physical, height, weight, and temperature are among the first tests your doctor will perform. The results may well provide the first indications of whether or not the general examination will conclude in a clean bill of health. Any abnormalities in these basic measurements may prompt the doctor to order additional laboratory work beyond the routine series of screening tests.

The reluctance of some doctors to discuss the details of test results with their patients often applies even to some of these basic measurements. There usually is no secret about your height and weight, even if the significance of changes in them may be unknown to you. If your temperature is normal, you will usually be informed. If it is abnormal, the doctor might hesitate to mention it. And when your pulse and blood pressure are taken, your questions may be rebuffed by a vague reply, such as "It's nothing to worry about"—as if it were none of your business and probably beyond your comprehension in any event.

Other doctors take the opposite approach. Not only do they freely discuss the results with you, but they sometimes frown and show displeasure in an attempt to shame you into improving your weight or blood pressure—if indeed they need improving—by changing your lifestyle. Fortunately, more doctors now recognize the motivational value to their patients of knowing, in terms of hard numbers, how they measure up physically and where they ought to be.

For example, if you are overweight and your blood pressure is a bit elevated, it may be possible to bring both within normal range without the need of any medication, just by cutting down on fatty foods and salt intake, eliminating cigarette smoking, and exercising regularly. But the motivation must be there. Without a specific goal, good intentions tend to be forgotten.

Today, increasingly more people keep track of their own basic measurements. Just a few years ago, for example, the only place you could buy a blood pressure machine—the tongue-twisting "sphygmomanometer"—was in a medical supply house with a doctor's prescription. Today, most pharmacies carry several different models, including electronic ones. People are learning how to use these machines and how to find and count the pulse in the wrist or neck. They know how much they should weigh for their body build. They know that these basic measurements can be every bit as important indicators of their health as any laboratory tests.

## Height

How can height be a possible indicator of malfunction or disease? After all, it is well recognized that how tall or short you happen to be is mainly a matter of heredity. Nor is it possible to make any valid generalizations about shorter people being less or more healthy than taller people. The answer is that what is important from the medical point of view is not the actual height, but the changes that may be observed between one examination and the next.

This is most obvious with children. Children grow. It is normal that a child's height change continuously. The annual measurements at school are taken to determine if such growth is following normal patterns. The latitude as to what is normal is quite wide, but it sometimes takes more than a parent's concern or approval to judge whether a child is growing at an acceptable rate.

Abnormal growth in children can be an indication of many types of organic deficiencies or diseases. These could include metabolic disorders in which the body cannot properly digest or utilize the nutrients in the diet; glandular abnormalities such as slow thyroid-gland function or diabetes mellitus; and, most commonly, any major illness of the kidneys. Pediatricians search carefully for such disorders if a child is seen because of "failure to thrive."

Excessive growth, which for a while seems to give the child an advantage over his or her contemporaries before turning into a disadvantage, can be caused by oversecretion of growth hormone by the pituitary gland. The cause of stunted growth usually is much harder to track down, often requiring extensive investigation and tests by the doctor. By uncovering the problem, the doctor may be able not only to restore normal growth, but also to correct some potentially life-threatening condition.

In adults, the problem is somewhat different simply because adults are not supposed to grow. What the doctor becomes concerned about in their case are signs of unexpected growth or shrinkage.

Even before measuring the patient's height and comparing it with that recorded on previous visits, a doctor may be alerted to excessive growth in adulthood, known as acromegaly. In this condition, the bones in the hands become disproportionately large; the jaw enlarges and begins to protrude; the tongue becomes enlarged and spaces may appear between the teeth. Actual height increase may occur in the bones of the spinal column. As with excessive growth in children, acromegaly is caused by oversecretion of growth hormone by the pituitary gland.

The loss of height can be equally dramatic. It is quite normal for older people to gradually lose as much as one inch in height due to changes in their posture or loss of bone substance related to the many factors involved in aging. What is abnormal is for younger people to rapidly lose height due to changes in the integrity of the skeleton. Such shrinkage can, over the years, amount to as much as three or four inches, particularly if fractures of the spinal vertebrae occur. This problem is usually caused by primary hyperparathyroidism, a condition that results from one or more overactive parathyroid glands. These glands are responsible for maintaining the body's calcium balance (page 67). When this system becomes overactive, it literally extracts calcium out of the bones, dissolves it in the bloodstream, and disposes of it in the urine, often causing kidney stones in the process.

Next time you are in a doctor's office, you should be aware that measuring your height as an adult is not as useless a part of the routine as you perhaps thought.

## Weight

Where do you find yourself in the tables of desired weight? (See page 21.) Are you within the normal range for your height and build? The normal ranges in these tables were determined the same way as normal ranges for various laboratory tests. They are based on a representative sample of our population that is considered to be healthy.

## DESIRABLE WEIGHTS FOR MEN AND WOMEN
## According to Height and Frame, Ages 25 and Over

| HEIGHT (In Shoes)* | Weight in Pounds (In Indoor Clothing) | | |
|---|---|---|---|
| | SMALL FRAME | MEDIUM FRAME | LARGE FRAME |
| **MEN** | | | |
| 5' 2" | 112-120 | 118-129 | 126-141 |
| 3" | 115-123 | 121-133 | 129-144 |
| 4" | 118-126 | 124-136 | 132-148 |
| 5" | 121-129 | 127-139 | 135-152 |
| 6" | 124-133 | 130-143 | 138-156 |
| 7" | 128-137 | 134-147 | 142-161 |
| 8" | 132-141 | 138-152 | 147-166 |
| 9" | 136-145 | 142-156 | 151-170 |
| 10" | 140-150 | 146-160 | 155-174 |
| 11" | 144-154 | 150-165 | 159-179 |
| 6' 0" | 148-158 | 154-170 | 164-184 |
| 1" | 152-162 | 158-175 | 168-189 |
| 2" | 156-167 | 162-180 | 173-194 |
| 3" | 160-171 | 167-185 | 178-199 |
| 4" | 164-175 | 172-190 | 182-204 |
| **WOMEN** | | | |
| 4' 10" | 92- 98 | 96-107 | 104-119 |
| 11" | 94-101 | 98-110 | 106-122 |
| 5' 0" | 96-104 | 101-113 | 109-125 |
| 1" | 99-107 | 104-116 | 112-128 |
| 2" | 102-110 | 107-119 | 115-131 |
| 3" | 105-113 | 110-122 | 118-134 |
| 4" | 108-116 | 113-126 | 121-138 |
| 5" | 111-119 | 116-130 | 125-142 |
| 6" | 114-123 | 120-135 | 129-146 |
| 7" | 118-127 | 124-139 | 133-150 |
| 8" | 122-131 | 128-143 | 137-154 |
| 9" | 126-135 | 132-147 | 141-158 |
| 10" | 130-140 | 136-151 | 145-163 |
| 11" | 134-144 | 140-155 | 149-168 |
| 6' 0" | 138-148 | 144-159 | 153-173 |

*1-inch heels for men and 2-inch heels for women.

SOURCE: October 1977 issue of Statistical Bulletin. Reprinted by permission of the Metropolitan Life Insurance Company.

As in laboratory tests, there might be a number of reasons why your weight could be outside the normal range. You might have weighed yourself after a particularly heavy meal. If you are a woman, unexpected weight gain may be an early sign of pregnancy. As a man, you may be exceptionally muscular with a Mr. Universe build. On the other hand, you might be just plain overweight!

How much do you worry if your weight is abnormal? Here you are on much more familiar ground than with laboratory tests. There is little of that mystery in checking your weight that there is in taking a blood or urine specimen. The terminology is both simple and familiar. You may be a bit concerned if your weight is outside the normal limits—but not as worried as when laboratory tests are abnormal. Yet your abnormal weight could be an indicator of a more serious problem than the abnormal lab test. The point is that a weight abnormality can be viewed in the same perspective as an abnormality in a lab test. Both require interpretation.

In checking on weight, the doctor is interested not only in how much you weigh, but how your latest weight compares with what you weighed in years past. If your lifestyle has remained unchanged, any loss or gain must have been caused by some factor which the doctor intends to pinpoint.

For example, the weight gain could be the result of edema, which is the overfilling of body tissues with water, often visible around the ankles. Edema could be indicative of a liver, heart, or kidney disorder. But in women, a two- or three-pound weight gain due to fluid is not unusual toward the end of the menstrual cycle. Some women associate this water retention with symptoms of irritability or so-called premenstrual tension.

An unexplained loss in weight, especially in the case of children, could be the first sign of diabetes. In fact, glandular disorders can cause unusual weight losses as well as unusual weight gains.

Diet, of course, is the main cause of a change in weight, and in our society the most frequent abnormality is overweight. A few years ago, most doctors rarely commented on an individual's weight, treating it as a personal matter that had no bearing on the physical examination. In some circles, overweight was considered a sign of well-being and prosperity. Many doctors had a similar portly appearance and were not in a position to preach self-improvement.

Today, doctors are increasingly conscious of their patients' weight. Current indications are that to be overweight is hazardous to one's health. Evidence is mounting on the relationship between obesity and higher incidence of heart attacks, arterial disease, and other degenerative disorders. Very often, just by losing weight, the patient may be able to substantially reduce these risks—and correct laboratory test abnormalities such as early diabetic blood sugar levels.

To be thin is becoming highly desirable in our society, and from the medical point of view, that is all for the better. Yet some people, especially young girls, may develop a severe illness in their desire to become thin. The condition known as anorexia nervosa is marked by virtually a total rejection of food, with weight losses that turn the individual into a veritable walking skeleton. Sometimes, death from malnutrition may result. It usually takes years of specialized counseling to overcome the condition.

Whatever your weight, it is more than just a matter of how you look. Often, it can be the key to your health.

## Temperature

Do you know what your normal temperature is? Practically every man, woman, and child knows that normal temperature is supposed to be 98.6° Fahrenheit. Yet, do you remember ever having precisely that temperature?

Depending on age, sex, and personal differences, temperature can vary somewhat and still be normal. For some people, it can be higher in the morning and lower in the evening—or vice versa. For children, temperature fluctuations are likely to be more pronounced than for adults. For women, temperatures may vary depending on the phase of their monthly menstrual cycle; a slightly elevated temperature generally signals ovulation. Some couples may use this phenomenon to avoid pregnancy; others may use it to promote conception.

An elevated temperature is one of the most common signs of disease, ranging from a common cold to lymph-gland tumors.

People often regard fever as a kind of disease in itself rather than a symptom of disease. Extreme fever of over 103° is in itself dangerous because of the risk of seizures and even brain damage. Fever should never be treated as an isolated disorder without finding the explanation for its origin.

Actually, fever usually should be regarded as one of the first lines of defense against bacterial infections. The rise in temperature is triggered by increased white cell activity in response to infectious agents.

When white blood cells do battle with these foreign invaders of your body, a class of proteins known as pyrogens are released and activate the temperature control mechanism deep within the brain.

The way your body temperature becomes elevated is a complex process. For one thing, the blood vessels near the surface of the skin become constricted, thereby reducing the amount of blood flowing through them that gets cooled by contact with the air. This may cause you to shiver, creating still more heat. At the same time, the body begins to burn up more energy, producing still more heat that is concentrated within you. For every degree of fever, your body uses 7 percent more energy. That is why you may actually lose weight when you are home in bed with a temperature, even though you do not move around as much as usual.

We have yet to learn exactly how a fever does its job. One line of thinking has it that high fever kills many of the invading bacteria and viruses which cannot tolerate the high temperatures to the same degree as other cells in the body. There is also evidence that fever may interfere with the invaders' ability to live off the nutrients in the body, especially iron. Moreover, fever speeds up the activity of white blood cells, letting them get to work faster and more effectively.

No matter how fever does its job, it *does* do it well. Without fever, many kinds of infections probably would be much more deadly than they are.

## Pulse

As a diagnostic tool, the pulse in recent years has come to be viewed with renewed interest. People with an active concern for their health often regard the pulse rate as one of the most simple and accurate indicators of their condition. Not only can the pulse serve as a built-in warning sign for many diseases, it can even be used to identify possible allergens in the diet and environment.

The pulse is basically a reflection of your heartbeat. It tells you how fast your heart is beating, how steadily, and how forcefully. The wrist is where the pulse usually is taken, although there are other points on the body, such as the throat and ankle, where the heart's pulsation can be felt especially well. These sites may prove useful when the blood pressure is too low to detect a pulse in the wrist.

A normal pulse is considered to be between 60 and 90 beats per minute. However, if you have rushed to your doctor's office, if you are worried about the examination, or if you have just enjoyed a substantial meal, do not be surprised if your pulse is considerably higher. Exercise, emotional stress, and eating all tend to raise the pulse temporarily.

Many health-conscious people measure their pulse to determine whether they are getting enough exercise. Some authorities on cardiovascular fitness believe that for the healthy heart to perform adequate work, a pulse rate in excess of 140 should be sustained for several minutes. How quickly the pulse then returns to normal is another indicator of your general physical condition.

People who exercise a lot tend to develop far lower pulse rates than the general population. Joggers or long-distance runners often have pulse rates as low as 45 per minute. This is considered to be a sign of good conditioning. Although beating less often than the heart of a person with a normal pulse of 70, the heart of an athlete is doing the same amount of work. The athlete's heart has become more efficient than the normal heart.

Some authorities believe that what is considered a normal pulse is in itself somewhat elevated. They suggest that people interested in good health should try to lower their pulse into the 60s. This can usually be done through regular exercise and other lifestyle changes.

Among such changes are elimination of foods or habits that tend to elevate the pulse unduly. For instance, if your pulse goes up after smoking, your pulse rate will be lowered by giving up smoking. Or if your pulse goes up after a couple of beers or exotic foods, moderating or avoiding the intake of these items also will help lower your pulse rate. Some people may be similarly sensitive to some non-exotic foods, such as bananas, milk, or bread.

But a slow pulse is not always a sign of vibrant good health. It might mean an underactive thyroid gland; if so, this could be determined by various thyroid tests. A very slow pulse could also result from taking medication, such as propanolol for high blood pressure or chronic headaches. Some tranquilizers also will induce a slow, steady pulse.

Periodic, sustained slowing of the pulse can be caused by changes in the natural rhythm of the heart. This potentially troublesome condition can be confirmed by an electrocardiogram, taken during a slow period, or by a twenty-four hour recording made by a portable cardiogram.

An excessively rapid pulse rate of over 100 beats per minute could be caused by an overactive thyroid gland or such conditions as arthritis, fever, or unrecognized heart disease. Follow-up laboratory tests, combined with other diagnostic tools available to the physician, usually will pinpoint the source of the trouble.

If the doctor suspects heart disease, the pulse may provide another clue in the form of skipped or added beats; these can readily be felt as sudden bumps in the pulse. On the other hand, some perfectly healthy people may occasionally have either skipped or added beats with no disease implications whatsoever. An electrocardiogram usually will tell your doctor whether the condition is anything to watch.

Taking your own pulse is not difficult and certainly can be a useful tool in assessing and improving your health. You can usually take your pulse by feeling, with the second and index fingertips of one hand, for the pulsation in the small artery of the wrist of your other hand. The number of pulsations you count in one minute is your pulse. But here, a word of caution. A person could become preoccupied with pulse-taking to such a degree that it becomes a kind of neurosis. Undue concern by itself may cause pulse irregularities which could aggravate a general state of hypochondriasis. Under those circumstances, pulse-taking would obviously become counterproductive and should be left to the medical and nursing professions at the appropriate time for checkups or other office visits.

## Blood Pressure

If you are over twenty-one, the chances are at least one in seven that you may have some form of high blood pressure, or hypertension. More than 20 million of our citizens have high blood pressure; about a third of them are unaware of it.

Knowing whether or not you have high blood pressure could help to save your life. The relationship between coronary heart disease and high blood pressure has been demonstrated repeatedly. Even borderline blood pressure elevations have been shown to increase complications of coronary heart disease by almost 50 percent. Yet, once you know that you do have it, most cases of high blood pressure can be well controlled with beneficial results in terms of health and longevity.

Measuring your blood pressure is an indispensible part of any physical examination. Even dentists frequently measure the patient's blood pressure before the work begins. Admittedly, a fearful patient with a sore tooth may have higher blood pressure than is customary. So do not panic if that is the case. Have your blood pressure taken again under more relaxed circumstances.

Free blood pressure clinics are often sponsored by communities, civic organizations, schools, and employers. There are even blood pressure machines in many shopping centers where you can make the measurement yourself for as little as fifty cents.

Making a precise blood pressure measurement is not always a simple matter. Depending on the circumstances, your blood pressure can vary considerably. Such factors as your emotional state, physical exercise, time of day, whether or not you have recently eaten or engaged in sexual activity can all affect the measurement. That is why reading outdated magazines while you sit in your doctor's waiting room may not be a complete waste of time. (If, on the other hand, you have another appointment soon after, you may become impatient, and then your blood pressure will rise.)

What the doctor is looking for is a general trend in your blood pressure over a period of years, and for any change from your usual pattern. If there is a change, your blood pressure will be taken again in several positions—sitting up, lying down, and standing—to confirm the reading.

Blood pressure refers to the force with which blood pushes against the walls of your major blood vessels. It is measured by a sphygmomanometer, an instrument with a soft cuff that is applied to the upper arm. The cuff is inflated by squeezing a rubber bulb until the pressure in the cuff becomes equal to the pressure in the main artery and briefly stops the blood flow. As the air is slowly released, the flow resumes and loud beats are heard in the artery by listening through a stethoscope applied just below the cuff.

When the first beat is heard, the reading on the pressure gauge represents the systolic pressure. Systolic pressure measures the peak force of the blood at the instant immediately after each beat of your heart.

The second, and lower, measurement is the force of the blood against your blood vessels when the heart is resting between beats. When the pressure in the cuff reaches this point, the sound of each heartbeat becomes only faintly audible. Suddenly, the sounds cease altogether, as the flow becomes continuous since the blood can now move freely through the artery. The blood pressure reading at the moment of this change in sound is known as the diastolic pressure.

Thus, your blood pressure reading consists of two numbers, representing your systolic and diastolic pressures. Using the metric system, each number represents the millimeters of mercury in a vertical column that are needed to balance the pressure in the cuff. If you are unclear as to exactly what that means, no matter. Understanding the numbers in terms of normal values is what is important.

What is normal? Again, this takes some interpretation. Generally, pressures up to 140 systolic and 90 diastolic—written 140/90 and read "one hundred and forty over ninety"—are considered within the normal range, with 140/90 to 160/95 being borderline. Anything over that is definitely high. Advancing age is an important factor, since a gradual rise over the decades normally is expected. It is the comparison to the normal trend that generally enables the doctor to make the correct interpretation of your reading.

The lower your blood pressure, the longer you are likely to live— provided, of course, your blood pressure stays within certain limits. The lower limit is not easily defined and can vary from individual to individual. Generally, pressures which continuously remain lower than 90/60 are suspect, and further tests are in order. Among the causes of abnormally low blood pressure, or hypotension, are anemia, low thyroid function, heart disorders, and iron deficiency. The term "tired blood" does have some meaning when it refers to these problems.

High blood pressure is not a disease in itself, but a sign of conditions affecting the blood vessels, kidneys, or adrenal glands. When there is permanent constriction of the blood vessels, it becomes necessary for the heart to work harder in doing its job of pumping blood throughout the body.

All of the causes of high blood pressure are not yet fully known. Among the common suspected factors are hereditary predisposition, protracted emotional stress, excessive intake of salt, and exposure to certain trace minerals, such as cadmium or nitrates in your food or water supply. Excessive secretion of a kidney hormone known as renin and overproduction by the adrenal glands of the salt-retaining hormone, aldosterone, have also been implicated in some forms of high blood pressure.

Hypertension has often been called the silent killer. Although symptoms may sometimes include shortness of breath, nosebleeds, headaches, and dizziness, at other times there are no symptoms whatsoever. The patient may feel perfectly fine, with no inkling that he or she may be close to physical disaster.

If untreated, high blood pressure can cause damage throughout the body. It can lead to both arteriosclerosis (a hardening of the outer walls of the medium-size arteries) and atherosclerosis (a buildup of fatty deposits on the inner surface of main-artery walls). It can lead to an enlarged heart and heart attack; rupture of delicate blood vessels in the retina of the eyes and blindness; permanent brain damage; and fatal kidney damage.

On detecting high blood pressure, the doctor will order additional lab tests, known as a hypertension profile. This series of tests includes measuring the blood levels of renin and aldosterone, salt and potassium, the blood urea nitrogen, and the urine output of adrenaline-type hormone products. The results enable the physician to narrow down the possible causes of high blood pressure, to prescribe the most appropriate treatment, and to discover if the patient has a curable form of this illness.

About 5 to 10 percent of patients who have high blood pressure for a very specific reason fall into the curable category. Typical examples of disorders which often can be cured permanently if diagnosed in the reversible stage of high blood pressure are tumors of the adrenal gland, an overactive thyroid gland, tumors capable of secreting adrenaline compounds, pituitary tumors producing either ACTH or growth hormone, and localized blood-flow constrictions in a main artery to one kidney. For this reason, it is best to have a hypertension profile early rather than late, since hypertension in these cases is a symptom of other, possibly fatal disorders.

Although there is no cure for all types of high blood pressure, treatment usually is effective in keeping it close to, or even within, the normal range. Such treatment involves a combination of diet, relaxation, and medication.

To determine the proper level of medication, the doctor may sometimes request the patient to buy a sphygmomanometer and take several blood pressure measurements each day at home. The readings in the relaxed atmosphere of one's home are likely to be lower than those obtained under the relatively stressful conditions of an office visit. The type of medication and dosage can then be adjusted for the best possible control of each individual case. And control, in most cases of high blood pressure, is what saves lives.

# 4
# Testing Your Urine

The testing of urine, or urinalysis, is perhaps the most common and certainly one of the simplest of all laboratory procedures. To obtain a sample involves none of the unpleasantness of a needle—even if some people are still a bit shy about handing over a bottle of their own bodily fluid. Be that as it may, many of us probably engage in some kind of basic urinalysis every time we go to the bathroom. How much urine is there? What color is it? Does it have an odor? We are not likely to consciously notice our own monitoring so long as we are healthy and our urine is normal. But should our urine suddenly turn a peculiar color, give off an unusual odor, or come forth in excessive quantities, we probably would notice right away.

The ready availability of a body sample is perhaps why urinalysis is one of the oldest of all medical testing procedures. Even 2,400 years ago, the pupils of Hippocrates were taught to study urine as a basis for predicting the course of each illness. At about the same time in another part of the world, the Hindu physician Sasruta was among the first to recognize the sweet taste of diabetic urine—a test that was still being used at the turn of this century by some general practitioners in the United States. Today, urinalysis is an infinitely more scientific procedure. Yet it remains simple enough that virtually anyone can perform many of the key tests with a minimum of training.

## What Kind of Disease Is It?

Rudimentary though his methods, Hippocrates knew that urinalysis could reveal events that occurred outside the urinary tract. The father of our medical profession taught his followers to examine urine as a way of finding out what was happening throughout the patient's entire body.

The same principle applies today. Urinalysis is similar to examining a sample from the mouth of a river in order to identify chemicals and other toxic products derived from sources upstream.

Emptying the bladder is a natural function for removing surplus quantities of water, salts, and countless waste products of digestion and metabolism. If something is wrong with our digestion or metabolism, the composition of the various waste products in the urine will alert us. Or the problem may be more specific, relating directly to the kidneys or other parts of the urinary tract.

The kidneys directly control the composition of urine by acting as filters. Over 1,500 quarts of blood flow through our kidneys each day. The various waste products from the body's tissues circulate in our blood, and it is up to the kidneys to filter them out.

Much of the material filtered out of the blood is reabsorbed in the kidneys and returned to the blood to maintain the proper balance of essential components in our body fluids. It is only the waste products—surplus water, excess sugar, and other constituents not necessary for the proper balance of blood chemistry—that are eliminated in this process.

In urine from normal persons, the exact chemical composition may vary, depending on their dietary intake and the body's metabolic activity. For example, the amount of sodium and chloride in your urine is directly related to how much salt you use. Another waste product is urea, which is a normal by-product of protein breakdown, such as from digestion of a hamburger. People on high-protein diets are likely to have higher levels of urea in their urine.

Other chemicals normally found in urine are the amino acids, which are the building blocks of proteins; enzymes, such as amylase, which are involved in the process of digestion; and hormones, reflecting the status of the body's glandular system. It is also common to find vitamins in the urine, particularly vitamin C, representing the daily excess in our food or supplements above the needs of the body.

## Initial Screening Examination

The routine urinalysis does not try to measure all the wastes in our urine. There are literally hundreds of such wastes that have already been identified, and the list is still growing. The initial screening examination is confined to identifying or measuring a select few which have a special meaning for the physician.

These are albumin, glucose, ketones, blood, and bile. Also checked in this initial screening is the pH, which is the relative acidity or alkalinity of the urine. The entire procedure is done in a few moments by dipping a plastic strip coated with chemicals into the urine sample and comparing the changes in the colors of these testing chemicals with a reference color chart. Testing strips are readily available in pharmacies for home use under special circumstances; for example, by persons with diabetes.

You may be surprised at first by the number of diseases any single abnormality may indicate. Keep in mind the fact that the physician makes a judgment on the basis of a complete physical examination and a variety of other tests, as well as some specialized follow-up tests.

## pH

The basic purpose of a pH test is to find out how acid or alkaline your urine is. This test is similar to the litmus paper test done in high school chemistry classes.

The relative degree of acidity or alkalinity of any solution is measured by pH. The pH range varies from 0 to 14, with 7 as neutral. A urine pH above 10 is extremely alkaline; below 3, very acid. Urine pH for normal adults is usually about 6.

Diet strongly affects the pH value of urine. If you eat large quantities of meat, other proteins, and even cranberries, your urine will become more acid. On the other hand, if your diet includes large amounts of vegetables or citrus fruits, your pH is likely to rise above 6. There is no hard-and-fast rule as to what your pH should be. Depending on what you eat, a consistent reading anywhere from 5.0 to 6.5 can be considered normal. Occasional results as low as 4.5 or as high as 7.5 are acceptable, but alert the physician to possible problems. For instance, very alkaline urine may result from infection due to formation of ammonia from urea by the enzymes of certain bacterial species.

Awareness of urine pH can be very useful for patients who suffer from kidney stones. If the stones are of the uric acid variety, it is important to keep the urine alkaline. If the stones contain much calcium, the urine should be kept acid. Uric acid stones are less likely to form in an alkaline medium, and calcium stones are less likely to form in an acid medium.

Extremely acid or extremely alkaline urine may be a sign of disturbances in the body's acid–alkali balance. In such cases, the urine pH may change to reflect the adjustment actions of the kidneys. When excess acids are formed or retained in the body to cause an acid condition, an acid urine is produced. The opposite can occur due to formation or retention of alkali in the two conditions known as metabolic alkalosis and respiratory alkalosis. In such cases, the urine produced is extremely alkaline.

Since either acidosis or alkalosis can be serious, the physician usually will call for further tests on any urine sample with an unusual pH value.

## *Albumin/Protein*

The test for albumin is also known as a test for protein, since albumin is the most common protein to be released into the urine.

You may already be familiar with the term "albumin" as a component of the white of an egg. Albumin in urine forms a clear solution similar to raw egg white. If heat is applied, albumin in urine changes into a solid substance, much like when egg white is cooked.

Until chemical tests were developed, the test for albumin consisted of heating the urine specimen in a test tube over a gas flame. If albumin was present, a cloudy material formed. This was far from convenient, considering the tendency of urine to froth, boil over, and release ammonia fumes. Today, a reagent test strip does a more accurate job in seconds and with no mess. More exact measurements for identifying the precise amount and type of protein are available if a positive test is found.

Even if your urine is normal, small amounts of protein may be present because certain molecules, such as albumin, can pass through the kidney's filtration membranes. Some of the urinary proteins also come from the prostate and seminal vesicles of the adult male. It is not uncommon to temporarily find protein in the urine after severe exercise, exposure to cold, or during an ordinary fever.

Any persistent elevation of urinary protein, however, may indicate significant kidney or lower-urinary-tract disease. The protein elevation may be the result of inflammation or breakdown of the kidney cell membranes which filter materials from the blood. When this occurs, large protein particles can enter the urinary tubules and pass into the urine.

Elevated protein frequently is seen in patients with such conditions as infections, high blood pressure, congestion of the renal veins due to heart failure, diabetic complications of the kidneys, a variety of chemical poisonings which can cause kidney damage, and a connective-tissue disease known as systemic lupus erythematosis.

If there definitely is protein in your urine, the physician has to evaluate and rule out many possibilities before a final conclusion can be reached. Additional tests for infection, X-ray studies of the kidneys, and studies of other organ functions may be needed to solve the problem.

## Glucose/Sugar

The primary reason for testing your urine for glucose is to detect whether or not you have sugar diabetes.

In normal individuals, a certain level of blood sugar is essential for maintaining life. The sugar in your blood is filtered within your kidneys, and, provided your glucose levels are normal, most of it is returned to your bloodstream before it can be excreted in the urine.

However, there is just so much sugar that the kidneys can handle. When the level of blood sugar exceeds this threshold, the kidneys' reabsorption mechanism is unable to handle the excessive load. Result? Sugar spills over into the urine. The amount of sugar spilled may be large enough to carry excess fluid with it, causing frequent urination as well as much thirst.

Sugar also may appear in the urine of non-diabetics. This condition is found in people whose kidneys for various reasons cannot reabsorb the normal amounts of sugar which they have filtered out. Patients with liver damage, brain injury, and various glandular problems, such as an overactive thyroid gland, also may have sugar in their urine.

Sugar in the urine may appear under certain conditions and yet be quite normal. If you eat large amounts of carbohydrates shortly before a sugar test, your result could show positive. You may also get a false positive result if you have taken large amounts of vitamin C or certain types of antibiotics prior to the test, because they interfere with chemical tests for sugar.

If, on the other hand, you consume large amounts of fluids prior to a urine test, your urine sugar may be diluted and the test show a negative result. For these reasons, a specimen taken before you eat or drink anything is more reliable than one taken afterward.

To eliminate or confirm the possibility of diabetes when a sugar test shows positive, more extensive tests such as glucose tolerance studies may have to be done under controlled conditions in which both the blood and urine are tested for sugar (see page 44).

A key purpose of the simple glucose test, done with a reagent strip dipped in urine, is to help diabetics adjust their diet and insulin dosage. By doing this test once or more each day in the privacy of their home, they are able to judge the safety of sugar levels in their system and make adjustments, if necessary, in their diet or medication.

## Ketones

Ketones are chemicals that appear in urine as the by-products of incomplete metabolism of fats. If you change to a low-calorie diet, your body will draw on its fat reserves to supply the needed energy. As your fat stores become depleted and you lose weight, a certain amount of ketones will accumulate in your blood and spill over into your urine.

The simple reagent-strip test for ketones has been widely popularized in connection with various low-carbohydrate diets. At times, there have been virtual runs on pharmacies, totally depleting normal supplies of the reagent-coated strips. A physician can use this same technique to learn whether a patient has been sticking to a weight reduction program well enough to cause fatty tissue to break down—or has been cheating.

Ketone tests, however, are not for dieters only. Finding ketones in the urine is one way of confirming diabetes. Ketones might also be found following anesthesia or frequent vomiting, and occasionally after severe stress, such as exposure to cold or very strenuous exercise. Because the body may not have sufficient sugar to provide the necessary energy under those conditions, it must again rely on its fat reserves. Ketones in the urine in these circumstances can be quite normal and need be no cause for concern.

## Hemoglobin/Blood

Testing for blood in the urine should be done promptly after the collection of the sample. If allowed to stand for any considerable time, the red blood cell membranes will break down and make measurement impossible.

You could have up to 1,000 red blood cells in every milliliter of urine and still be normal with no cause for concern. These cells usually come from the urinary tract and bladder, and result from the normal leakage of a few cells here and there. This normal leakage of red blood cells is not enough to give a positive chemical test for hemoglobin, the red-colored substance responsible for oxygen transport in the blood.

A far greater amount of hemoglobin, sufficient to show up as a positive result, could indicate kidney problems: kidney stones, a tumor, inflammation, or damage to the tissues that filter the bloodstream. These changes can be detected by the microscope long before the urine would change color when larger quantities of red cells were released.

### Bilirubin/Bile

If you want to understand what it means to have bilirubin in the urine, it is essential to first read the section on bilirubin as a blood constituent (page 52). This is because too much bilirubin in the blood is what gives rise to too much bilirubin in the urine.

As with abnormal amounts of bilirubin in the blood, a positive finding in the urine indicates there may be problems with the liver or the bile excretory system. Or there may be an increased destruction of red cells in the blood, in the condition known as hemolytic anemia.

A positive urine result for bilirubin should be followed up with specific blood and other tests to determine precisely whether the cause is related to the liver, to the bile excretory system, or to an increased breakdown of red blood cells.

## Physical Characteristics

When your urine specimen is subjected to a routine examination, additional observations are made as a way of finding other potential disorders within your body. The reagent-strip test takes just a few moments. After this, the urine will be subjected to a microscopic examination; it also will undergo a special test to determine its specific gravity; and it will be closely scrutinized for any unusual appearance, discoloration, or other notable physical characteristics.

Here, a word of caution. Although you yourself may be fully capable of making these observations, it takes training to make the proper evaluations—and these often have to be confirmed by further specialized testing.

The normal appearance of urine can vary from pale to dark yellow, depending on the amount of fluid intake. The darker the urine, the more concentrated it is. The darker urine is usually caused by a decreased amount of fluid intake or because there has been a fluid loss due to sweating, vomiting, or diarrhea.

If the urine has an unusual color, you should consider the effects of certain foods, drugs, or candies which you may have eaten. The dyes in candies, as well as in certain other foods, can discolor urine. But there are few hard-and-fast rules. For example, the consumption of rhubarb can give a brown color to the urine if the urine is acid. In alkaline urine, rhubarb in the diet will result in an orange color. Beets can give a reddish color and carrots a yellow color to urine.

When the unusual color cannot be attributed to diet or drug therapy, then other factors may have to be investigated. If the urine is yellow-orange or even orange-brown, the color may be the result of fever or dehydration. Or it may be that the urine contains increased amounts of bilirubin substances, which could be a tip-off to liver, bile duct, or blood disorders.

A red or red-brown color is commonly seen in abnormal urine, and may indicate the presence of blood or hemoglobin. Red blood cells in the urine raise the possibility of some kind of kidney problem or urinary-tract infection. Stones or even tumors are other possible causes of blood in the urine. In menstruating women, care has to be taken not to contaminate the urine sample. The use of a tampon before the specimen is collected is recommended. It may be best to wait a few days until the blood flow has subsided.

Brownish-red urine is seen when a substance called myoglobin is excreted. Myoglobin is derived from muscle tissue. In situations of severe muscle cramps, excessive exercise, or trauma, myoglobin may be released into the bloodstream and then eliminated in the urine. Large quantities of myoglobin in the urine may be an early warning signal of excessive breakdown of skeletal muscle.

Brown-red urine may also be indicative of certain types of porphyria. The term "porphyria" covers a group of disorders in the chemical processes involved in the production of hemoglobin molecules. A genetic class of disease, it sometimes assumes such bizarre signs as a reddish glow of the gums and a peculiar sheen in the face. It is believed that some of the European werewolf legends were based on those unfortunates who, in fact, had porphyria. Another suspected porphyria sufferer: King George III, whose periodic bouts of "madness" may well have been attacks of porphyria, which is associated with mental derangement as well as abdominal pains, constipation, and other local nervous symptoms.

When normal urine is allowed to cool from body temperature, a white crystalline sediment consisting usually of phosphates and urate crystals becomes visible. Again, these are usually normal by-products of diet. You may also see small, cloudy precipitates, which are formed from the mucus of the urinary or genital tract. This is also normal.

Cloudy urine, however, may also result from the presence of white blood cells and various bacteria. This indicates some type of inflammation or infection of the urinary tract.

If sufficient bacteria are present, the urine may have the unpleasant smell of ammonia. Although other odors may be diet-related, such as from eating asparagus, some of these odors might also be genetically caused. Genetically caused odors of the urine tend to be musty or sweet, as for example, "maple sugar urine disease." Its characteristic odor results from the body's inability to utilize all the amino acids in such protein foods as meat and milk. It is the unused amino acids, or their by-products, which cause the unpleasant odor.

Finally, here is a simple test you can do yourself if you suspect you may have bladder or urinary tract infection. Empty the entire contents of your bladder into a glass container. If the urine is at all cloudy or if you see any particles floating in it, take some household vinegar and pour enough of it into the urine until the cloudiness disappears. Then watch for any stringy particles. If they remain floating, they are merely undissolved mucus and you are probably well. If, however, some of them plummet to the bottom of the glass, or if some are already resting on the bottom, then it is time to see your doctor.

## Microscopic Examination

The examination of urine sediment under a microscope is a routine part of urinalysis, and can provide further clues to the diagnosis of kidney disease. The sediment is obtained by spinning a random sample of urine in a centrifuge. The type of substances to look for in urine sediment are cells—red, white, and epithelial—casts, crystals, and various amorphous materials.

*Red blood cells,* which circulate throughout the bloodstream carrying oxygen to each tissue, can appear in the urine sediment during certain types of abnormal conditions. Very few red blood cells will be seen in the sediment if your urine is normal. If more than a small number are observed under a microscope, there may be a source of bleeding in the kidneys or the lower urinary tract. Injuries, tumors, infections, tissue damage, blood clot formation, or toxic drug reactions within the kidneys can cause an abnormal leakage of red blood cells into the urine. Their presence alerts the physician to search for one of these explanations.

*White blood cells,* called leukocytes, are occasionally found in a normal urine sediment under a microscope. Females may have slightly more leukocytes than males and still be within the normal range. An increased amount of white blood cells in kidney diseases is usually indicative of infection or some type of inflammatory process. Bladder tumors, prostatitis, urethritis, and urinary tract infections may also produce leukocytes in increased numbers. If your doctor suspects an infection, a urine culture should be performed to isolate and identify the bacteria causing the problem and to test their sensitivity to various antibiotics. If your urine specimen is not fresh, the presence of leukocytes may be missed altogether. Like red blood cells, leukocytes are delicate and can disintegrate as the urine stands at room temperature.

*Epithelial cells* are specialized cells which cover the surface of the body, its canals, tubules, and other organic structures. There may be occasional epithelial cells in your urine sediment as a result of the normal shedding process within the urinary tract. However, larger amounts of epithelial cells may indicate inflammatory changes or degeneration of kidney cells.

*Casts* can be found only in fresh urine sediment. These gelatin-like structures, made up of protein material, may also contain various cells or tiny crystals. If your urine sediment is normal, it is unlikely to contain any casts. This is because casts usually form when the kidneys are diseased and allow protein materials to seep into the urine tubules from the bloodstream. It is from these upper kidney tubules that casts take their characteristic cylindrical shape. The presence of many casts is indicative of serious kidney problems, requiring further investigation.

*Crystals* are materials of defined and specific shape that may bond together to form stones. They are formed by the precipitation of such substances as uric acid, cholesterol, bilirubin, amino acids, and various salts. If your urine is normal, there may be urate, oxalate, phosphate, carbonate, or uric acid crystals, depending on the acidity of the urine. Unusual types of crystals composed of tyrosine, leucine, or cystine are caused by disturbances of protein metabolism. Sulfonamide crystals may be seen following administration of sulfa drugs, unless large amounts of liquids are taken with that type of medication. Crystals can be recognized by their particular shapes and, when necessary, can be further identified by chemical tests.

Some persons may have all of these crystals in their urine sediment and never develop a stone. If the crystals are bonding together to form stones, it is helpful to strain the urine through cheesecloth to recover fragments of the stones for analysis of mineral and organic compounds.

From the composition of the stones, it frequently is possible to tell their cause, and this, in turn, leads to a plan for preventive treatment. Calcium and uric acid make up the major substances in urinary stones and require very different approaches in medication, diet, and control of the pH of the urine. Acid urine helps to prevent formation of calcium crystals; alkaline urine tends to dissolve uric acid crystals.

*Amorphous substances* may be found in a microscopic examination of the urine sediment. These are composed of materials similar to those in crystals, but lack a specific and definite shape. Amorphous substances require a special analysis to determine their nature. They may be the first warning of the start of the progression to crystals and eventual kidney stones.

---

*Specific gravity*
Normal range: 1.016 to 1.022

---

The specific gravity of urine is a measure of the amount of wastes consisting of salts and other body constituents that have been filtered out of the blood and now are removed in the urine. The test is not unlike measuring the specific gravity of an automobile battery to determine how good it is. But unlike the battery test—where the specific gravity can only be too low—the specific gravity of urine can either be too low or too high.

Measuring the specific gravity of your urine is another routine part of basic urinalysis. By this test, your doctor obtains an indication of kidney function, i.e., how well your kidneys are doing their job of filtering the blood; removing wastes, excess fluids, and salts; and returning vital constituents into the bloodstream in well-regulated quantities.

If the specific gravity of your urine has fallen below the normal range, the chances are that you are eliminating too much water, while many of the wastes, salts, and other constituents in your blood are not being removed. This causes a potentially toxic situation for your body.

If, on the other hand, you are eliminating too many salts and the specific gravity of your urine is above normal limits, some of the blood constituents that are being filtered out along with the wastes are not being properly reabsorbed and returned into your bloodstream. This could lead to a depletion or imbalance of the vital constituents in your bloodstream.

A test for checking the normal concentrating function of your kidneys can be done by withholding all fluids for at least sixteen hours, in which case it would be normal for the specific gravity of your urine to increase to 1.025 or greater.

Urine of low specific gravity need not mean kidney disease. It could be that the flow of urine has been increased by drinking coffee, which often has a natural diuretic effect. There is also a factor in the body known as antidiuretic hormone. People deficient in this hormone will produce copious amounts of urine low in specific gravity, even though their kidneys may be functioning just fine.

A hereditary form of this problem is caused by the failure of the kidneys to respond to the antidiuretic hormone. The condition is detected when fluid restriction does not stop fluid loss, and the patient becomes dehydrated and very thirsty. In such cases, the specific gravity of the urine can fall to 1.000, the same as tap water.

If the gravity reading is always below 1.005, the person is simply taking more fluids than are needed and will achieve higher readings when fluids are withheld. This condition is sometimes caused by compulsive water drinking. The affected person may have started the habit for obscure reasons, such as the belief that the kidneys need to be flushed to remove toxins. The original purpose is often forgotten. The person may try to replenish the fluids as fast as they are eliminated, and the waterlogged kidneys experience a loss of concentrating function. An enforced drying-out period will usually restore normal function as the body begins to manufacture the antidiuretic hormone again.

# 5
# Your Blood Chemistry Profile

You may not be aware of it, but the chances are that you probably have already had your blood analyzed for as many as a dozen very important components.

Your doctor may have ordered these tests as a routine part of your last complete physical examination. Unless the results turned up some striking abnormality, you were not even advised of the details. They would most likely have had very little meaning for you anyway.

Blood chemistry tests are ordered regularly by doctors to get a general indication of the body's health. During the onset of disease, subtle changes may occur in blood chemistry which are not detectable by any other procedures available to your physician.

What basically *is* blood chemistry testing? It is a very precise science of isolating various chemicals that are carried in the bloodstream in minute amounts. Blood chemistry is a matter of identifying them and finding out how much there is of each of them.

These chemicals are in your blood, but they are not visible under a microscope in the way red and white blood cells are. Literally hundreds of different chemicals have already been identified in the blood, and new ones are still being discovered.

The chemicals in your blood include various nutrients, carrying agents, catalysts, waste matter, and many other constituents whose role cannot be so neatly summarized, but whose presence is of vital importance to the proper functioning of your body.

Above all, *presence in the right amounts*. The amounts we are dealing with in these tests are, for the most part, minuscule. If isolated from a test tube of blood, most of these chemicals would be hardly visible

—and some would, indeed, be invisible to the naked eye. Yet, should their quantity increase or decrease by a small amount, it could spell serious trouble for the patient.

In explaining each test, there will be one guiding objective throughout this book: to enable you to understand what role each of the substances plays in making your body function smoothly. This approach should make it all the clearer as to what might go wrong with your body when these substances are not present in the proper amounts.

Here, a word of caution. All explanations will necessarily be in broad outlines, highlighting the main functions, the main interactions, the main physiological processes that may be affected by the substances under consideration. As intricate as some of these functions may seem, in reality they are invariably more complex. At any given moment, there are literally millions of reactions going on in your body, constantly affecting and influencing one another. No matter how long the book, it would be impossible to detail them all; many of them are not well understood, even by medical researchers. Modern science has yet to solve countless mysteries of how the human body does indeed work.

Obviously, it would be both impractical and unnecessary to test for all the hundreds of different constituents in your blood every time you have a physical. What your doctor may do is to choose a systematic approach, ordering a group of anywhere from twelve up to twenty-one different tests. These are done at a relatively low cost on an automatic machine called the autoanalyzer. They normally are more than sufficient to get an indication of any potential trouble. They give the doctor a chance to detect various diseases at a stage where the patient can still have the best chance to recover.

If the doctor has already zeroed in on the disease, the sharpshooter approach may be used, ordering far fewer but very specific tests. These will lead to a more accurate diagnosis and a more effective course of treatment. By ordering the same tests at periodic intervals throughout the illness, the physician will be able to monitor the patient's progress.

Included in this chapter are twenty-one of the most common blood chemistry tests. According to one estimate, some 6 billion tests are done each year in the United States at an approximate cost of $20 billion. In terms of frequency, the tests in this chapter represent perhaps half of all the testing procedures done on blood samples.

*Blood constituent: Glucose*
Normal range: 70 to 110 milligrams per 100 milliliters (mg/100 ml)

The test for glucose is one of the most basic and important of all laboratory tests. By measuring the sugar level in your blood, this test is useful in diagnosing diabetes as well as low blood sugar, or hypoglycemia.

Sugar is the basic fuel of the body in carrying out its normal functions, whether physical or intellectual. The American diet includes abundant sources of sugar; overabundant, some might say. These sources consist not only of such items as candies, pastries, and fruit but also such complex carbohydrates as bread and potatoes. The enzymes in saliva and in the small intestine break down these foods to their basic structure: glucose.

Glucose is readily absorbed into your bloodstream from the intestine. Sugar in pure form is taken up quickly, and within minutes supplies energy to the cells of your entire body. The more complex carbohydrates are broken down more gradually. That is why you may see sprinters munching on chocolate bars just before competing, while marathon runners will eat spaghetti, bread, and potatoes to store up glycogen and fat for days in advance of a contest.

The normal level for glucose usually means the fasting level and is referred to as the FBS, or fasting blood sugar. Following a meal heavy in sweets and other carbohydrates, it may be normal for the glucose level in your blood to briefly increase to 150–165 milligrams per 100 milliliters and return to the fasting level.

This rapid removal of blood glucose is the work of a hormone called insulin, secreted by the pancreas in response to the glucose increase. Although the specific, final action of insulin is not yet fully known, it is clear that insulin helps to move the glucose from the bloodstream into the body's cells and promotes the conversion of glucose to energy.

Insulin also stimulates the formation of glycogen, which is a multiple form of glucose suitable for storage in the body rather than for immediate use. Glycogen is made out of glucose that your body does not need to meet its present requirements. Stored primarily in the liver, glycogen is held in reserve for times when your muscle cells might require more energy than is available from blood glucose alone. Any glucose excess not needed for glycogen reserves ends up as fat—usually deposited around the midsection or the upper thighs.

Diabetes mellitus—or sugar diabetes or, simply, diabetes—is basically a condition of inadequate insulin secretion. The main purpose of analyzing your blood for glucose is to discover diabetes. If you are healthy, your glucose levels will remain in the normal range while fasting. If your supply of insulin is not sufficient, your fasting glucose levels will remain elevated. To confirm whether a single elevated glucose result is in fact due to diabetes, the physician will order what is known as a glucose tolerance test.

The glucose tolerance test requires that the patient consume, on an empty stomach, a premeasured amount of glucose—usually a fruit-flavored sugar solution. Blood specimens and urine specimens are then taken at regular intervals over the next three hours. The glucose will spill over into the urine whenever blood levels are greater than approximately 160 milligrams per 100 milliliters.

The purpose of measuring the different blood glucose levels at several intervals is to see exactly how well the ingested sugar is being taken up by the cells and how well the insulin is able to disperse it throughout the body. If the initial blood glucose prior to consumption of the sugar dose was elevated and if it remains elevated for more than two hours following the intake of the sugared drink, then some form of diabetes is indicated.

If the fasting blood sugar is normal but the tolerance test shows above-normal results, the condition is termed pre-diabetes and may represent an early stage of this disorder. Pre-diabetes can often be detected in individuals who have two parents that are diabetic. Such individuals should be tested periodically to diagnose this tendency to develop diabetes in order to institute protective dietary control before the disease becomes more serious.

There are almost four million known diabetics in the United States, with perhaps another two million as yet undiagnosed. Among juveniles, it is one of the most prevalent medical problems.

We are used to thinking of all diabetes cases as the usual hereditary form of diabetes mellitus. But there are other disorders which are known as causes of secondary diabetes. Lack of a family history of diabetes in near relatives may be a tip-off to such conditions as acromegaly (an excess of growth hormone), an overactive thyroid gland, liver malfunction, or overactive adrenal glands. Finding and correcting these causes may lead to a reversal of the diabetes. Your physician has access to many specific tests which can solve the mystery of secondary diabetes.

Sometimes a false alarm is generated by a positive urine test for glucose when the person is not diabetic. This is called renal glycosuria, which means that the kidneys are not able to reabsorb glucose when the blood glucose is even slightly above normal. Follow-up glucose tolerance tests reveal this situation and show normal blood sugar at times when urine tests show strongly positive reactions for sugar.

This finding is a great relief to the person but presents a problem whenever urine tests are done for insurance or health screening purposes. A copy of the glucose tolerance test results comes in handy for the affected individual to present to the examiner before the insurance application is reviewed.

What happens if your problem is not too much sugar in your blood, but not enough?

Low blood sugar, or hypoglycemia, is suspected when the fasting glucose level falls below 50 milligrams per 100 milliliters. To further determine whether a patient has hypoglycemia, the physician will order a glucose tolerance test, lasting from five to six hours, depending on the patient's history.

The procedure in this test is similar to that in the shorter test for diabetes except that the physician watches for a drop-off from the early high levels of glucose in the blood to the later low levels; how much of a spread occurs between the highest and the lowest levels; and how far the level might actually drop below the lower fasting limit before it returns to the fasting level.

For example, does the glucose level approach the fasting level in the second hour, the third hour, or later? Is the elevation in the first hour only minimal or does it reach into the diabetic range—as it well might? Does the lowest level fall only a few milligrams below fasting or does it dip as much as 15 milligrams?

There is considerable debate within the medical profession as to exactly what constitutes hypoglycemia. Some doctors maintain that too sudden a drop, too great a range between the high and low glucose levels, or any drop of more than 100 milligrams below peak levels—regardless of how high the fasting level—could constitute hypoglycemia and serve to generate symptoms of weakness or lack of energy. Individuals have different requirements, these doctors maintain, and the key to diagnosing hypoglycemia is to watch for some of the typical low-blood-sugar symptoms during any extended glucose tolerance test: nervousness, sweaty palms, dizziness, and even blackout spells.

How does hypoglycemia occur? If you are a healthy individual, when your blood glucose levels are approaching normal fasting levels perhaps a few hours after eating sweets, two things will happen. First, your insulin will shut off, thus reducing or stopping further removal of glucose from your bloodstream. Second, your liver will begin manufacturing new glucose—not from starches or carbohydrates, which have already been depleted, but from proteins. This glucose will find its way into your blood where it will replace any that is still being removed by whatever insulin may still be present.

The manufacture of glucose from protein and the inhibition of insulin secretion are both controlled by the adrenal gland hormone called cortisol. Hypoglycemia may be due to inadequate cortisol secretion, improper functioning of the liver or the pancreas, or a combination of all three. When excess insulin is observed in serious forms of hypoglycemia, the disease is also known as hyperinsulinism and may indicate the presence of an insulin-secreting tumor of the pancreas.

It is often said that many hypoglycemics in their thirties and forties become diabetics in their forties and fifties. The theory is that the prediabetic pancreas is slow to release its insulin and the delay causes high glucose followed by low glucose levels due to faulty timing. Eventually the pancreas can no longer secrete sufficient insulin, and the end result is diabetes mellitus.

Possibly the most common type of hypoglycemia is not a disease at all, but a disorder caused by dietary habits. At some time we are all guilty of consuming quick sources of food energy when we are busy or tempted by doughnuts, cookies, and the like. Taken with sugar-sweetened coffee or tea or a soft drink, the combination acts like a mini–glucose tolerance test. The abrupt rise in blood sugar triggers release of insulin, and the sugar supply is quickly used up. But enough insulin remains in the bloodstream to cause blood sugar to fall below normal.

Symptoms resembling an insulin reaction may occur, and the net effect may be a craving for more of the same foods. This aggravates the situation, since it provokes more insulin release, more rebound hypoglycemia, and greater craving for sweets. The glucose tolerance test reveals this form of hypoglycemia, known as reactive hypoglycemia, at three to five hours after starting the test.

If there is any doubt about the diagnosis, your doctor can order measurements of the actual amount of insulin in your blood. Such tests should indicate normal insulin levels while fasting and very low, even unmeasurable, insulin after the blood sugar has fallen below normal. This means that the fault is in the sources of sugar and not in the amount of insulin released.

The treatment? Strict avoidance of pure sugar, sweets, and high-carbohydrate foods. For energy, reliance is placed on frequent feedings of protein foods, including between-meal snacks. The affected person must cultivate a taste for cheese, eggs, fish, meat, poultry, peanut butter, and soybeans or soy products, all of which are high in protein.

It may seem strange to substitute a wedge of cheese for a slice of cake, but it moderates insulin release and provides a slowly released supply of glucose which offers a steady source of energy. In time, the jack rabbit release of insulin is lessened and the strict high-protein diet may be relaxed.

One other hint: Alcohol can act as a similar trigger for insulin. The antidote? Cheese and peanuts before cocktails. Try the dairy dip too, but watch out for the potato chips (carbohydrates again).

Whether testing for hypoglycemia or diabetes, the specimen must be protected with a special preservative to ensure that the blood will not clot and that the glucose will not actually be destroyed in the tube while awaiting analysis. If the test is to be performed on unpreserved blood, the clear serum must be separated from the blood cells soon after the specimen has clotted. Otherwise, the glucose will again be partly metabolized, giving a lower blood glucose level than actually exists within the body.

A new glucose test called glycohemoglobin has recently been reported to the public. It is used to assess long-term control of diabetic patients, especially children, who have erratic blood sugar patterns. Sustained elevations of blood glucose cause formation of glycohemoglobin, and its amount reflects months of exposure of the red blood cells to varying levels of glucose.

This certainly is an advance, but remember that diabetic control can already be assessed in many ways: by records of urine tests during the day; by twenty-four-hour spillage of sugar; by fasting blood sugar at each office visit; and by the state of health of each patient. The choice of tests is up to the physician. If the new test will help, it will be used; if not, remember that medical judgment is the basis for treatment; that tests provide a means to that end, but are not the be-all and end-all.

---

*Blood constituent: BUN*
Normal range: 10 to 25 milligrams per 100 milliliters (mg/100 ml)

---

BUN is the abbreviation for blood urea nitrogen. The test can be a tip-off for a number of disease conditions relating primarily to your kidneys. Excessive concentrations of BUN can be fatal.

BUN represents the end point of protein breakdown in your body. The first step in this process is the reduction of proteins to amino acids. These, in turn, are converted to carbon dioxide, water, and ammonia. Since ammonia is toxic to your body, it is converted by your liver to urea. And urea is dissolved in your blood, then carried to your kidneys, through which it is eliminated.

Urea is a small molecule, capable of penetrating cell membranes. Because of this ability, urea appears in saliva, perspiration, intestinal fluids, and even in the fluids within your brain and spinal cord.

Your level of BUN depends basically on three interrelated factors: the amount of protein you eat, your body's rate of protein breakdown —as determined by the various hormone regulators—and the ability of your kidneys to excrete urea as a waste product.

BUN levels in your blood may increase above normal if you become dehydrated. When this happens, there is a reduced flow within your kidneys, resulting in a proportionately higher amount of BUN being reabsorbed. The kidneys simply do not have a sufficient flow of urine to remove BUN efficiently from the bloodstream.

BUN levels may also increase if you are on a high-protein diet. It is a case of the more protein you take in, the more urea residue there is likely to be in your bloodstream.

Elevations in BUN can signify problems with the kidneys or within the entire urinary-tract system. An obstruction, such as kidney stones, might temporarily block urea elimination, increasing the chances of more urea being reabsorbed into the body. The decreased flow of fluid through the urinary tract also would not provide sufficient volume to flush out the waste urea. Other disease conditions that result in lowered blood flow to the kidneys, such as congestive heart failure or edema, also can cause elevated BUN levels.

Another cause of increased BUN is internal hemorrhage. When there is a rapid loss of blood, the volume of plasma decreases and the concentration of BUN in the blood rises correspondingly. Even after bleeding stops, the digestion of blood provides more protein for urea formation.

Infections, cancers, increased thyroid activity, uncontrolled sugar diabetes, or overaction of the adrenal glands can all lead to high BUN by causing an increased breakdown of various proteins in the body.

If the function of the kidneys becomes impaired, elimination of BUN becomes inadequate and a condition known as uremia develops.

Patients with kidney failure and uremia have greatly elevated BUN values, even in excess of 200 milligrams per 100 milliliters. The high

BUN indicates that other poisons are probably also accumulating in the blood. If this degree of BUN elevation continues for any period of time, coma or death will likely be the result. However, BUN and most of the other toxic products of the body are water-soluble, and artificial kidney dialysis is able to lower dangerous levels of these materials for two or more days between each treatment.

Subnormal levels of BUN are extremely rare and do not usually constitute a clinical problem. Severe protein malnutrition, water intoxication, and cirrhosis of the liver are some of the uncommon conditions that could give this type of result.

---

*Blood constituent: Creatinine*
Normal range: Less than 1 milligram per 100 milliliters (mg/100 ml)

---

The level of creatinine in your blood provides another very good indication of how your kidneys are working.

Creatinine is a waste material resulting from the breakdown of a substance called creatine phosphate. This substance interacts with other body substances to produce energy and, as this energy is used in making muscles work, creatinine is left behind as a waste product.

The formation of creatinine in your body remains rather constant. It does not vary with how much protein you eat, as is the case with BUN. Moreover, creatinine levels in your blood are unrelated to fluid intake or water balance.

Because of this independence from other factors, creatinine is very useful as an indicator of kidney function. If the creatinine level in your body remains within normal range, it is because your kidneys are functioning properly, filtering and excreting the necessary amounts of toxic wastes. If the creatinine level in the body exceeds the normal range, it is because the kidneys are unable to do their job and creatinine backs up in the blood.

Abnormal creatinine levels thus indicate either that the kidneys' ability to filter and remove waste from the bloodstream has been severely damaged or that there is a reduced blood flow to the kidneys caused by poor circulation or obstructing blood clots. An elevated level of creatinine is considered a serious prognostic sign indicating malfunction of both kidneys, since even one healthy kidney is enough to keep the level within normal limits.

---

*Blood constituent: Uric Acid*
Normal range, males: 2.5 to 8.5 milligrams per 100 milliliters
  (mg/100 ml)
Normal range, females: 2.5 to 6.5 milligrams per 100 milliliters
  (mg/100 ml)

---

The level of uric acid is typically elevated in a condition called gout. Gout involves a relatively large amount of uric acid being deposited in the vicinity of cartilage tissues. When microcrystals form in the fluids within joints, an acutely painful affliction occurs; this is called an attack of gout. The disease primarily affects males, and its incidence is thought to be family-related.

Gout is a disease that for centuries has often been made light of. Perhaps this is because gout was thought to affect portly men of high social stature who were suspected of overindulgence in rich food and alcohol. Among gout's more famous victims was Samuel Johnson, the great British dictionary-maker and man of letters, who not only chronicled the lives of many of his eighteenth-century contemporaries but described the progress of his own disease as well.

Gout is certainly nothing to joke about. It can be one of the most painful of all diseases. Among the first indications of gout is an unbearable soreness in the joints of the toes, especially the big toe. With progression of this disorder, uric acid is deposited even over the cartilage of the ear. You may be able to spot gout victims by the nodules along their outer ears.

How do people get gout? It is a metabolic disorder caused either by increased production of uric acid in the body or by decreased elimination of this material through the kidneys.

Uric acid is the end point in the breakdown of what are known as nucleic acids. Nucleic acids are complex molecules which store the genetic information needed to encode the individual characteristics of each cell. Nucleic acids are especially plentiful in such meats as liver and other organs. When components of the nucleic acids, called purines, are eliminated from body cells, they are converted by the liver into uric acid.

The kidneys filter uric acid and eliminate this organic waste into the urine. The amount of uric acid in the urine reflects the amount of purines that were broken down in the body. An excessive amount of uric acid in the urine can contribute to the formation of uric acid kidney stones, especially if the urine is highly acid. If stone formation takes place deep within the kidneys, serious damage can result.

A person's diet can influence the amount of uric acid produced to some extent. A physician may advise a patient suffering from gout to avoid foods rich in purines, such as the organ meats and various types of beans. Also, under starvation conditions, uric acid may become elevated because of the increased breakdown of tissue necessary to sustain life. Individuals with uric acid problems who want to diet seriously, therefore, have to be especially careful. It may be difficult for such persons to limit meat intake to under six ounces daily—no more than one typical hamburger or a roast beef sandwich. The standard combination of frankfurters and beans becomes a threat, and the search for the perfect chili must be abandoned.

But there is just so much that can be done to reduce uric acid levels through avoidance of dietary purines. Ultimately, gout is a metabolic disease. Uric acid production and its excretion by the kidneys occurs at an elevated rate even when the diet is relatively low in purines. So most physicians will prescribe medications which interfere with uric acid production or promote its excretion by the kidneys.

In addition to gout, uric acid elevations are common when the kidneys are not functioning properly; in essential hypertension, leukemia, and toxemia of pregnancy; and as a side effect of most diuretic drugs.

Subnormal levels of uric acid do not constitute a clinical problem. However, the latest medications for gout can prove so effective that production of uric acid may be depressed. Your physician is trained to adjust gout medication gradually until the elevated serum uric acid reaches normal limits. Periodic tests are taken to ensure adequate control and to avoid surprise attacks of gout. The pain of even one such episode is enough to instill respect for this simple laboratory test and the help it can give.

---

*Blood constituent: Bilirubin*
Normal range: Less than 1.2 milligrams per 100 milliliters (mg/100 ml)

---

The bilirubin test is a very useful for finding out if you have any disorders of the liver, bile ducts, or red blood cells.

Bilirubin is basically a waste product of the breakdown of hemoglobin, the oxygen-carrying portion of the red blood cells. Hemoglobin breakdown is a normal part of the constant process of regeneration and renewal throughout your body, some cells dying while others are being produced. Bilirubin is largely made up of the pigment of red blood cells that have died.

Bilirubin in this form is not soluble in water and cannot be eliminated in the urine. Known as indirect bilirubin, this waste product must first be carried by the bloodstream to the liver, where it will be made into a water-soluble form called direct bilirubin. As direct bilirubin, it can now be readily eliminated from your body in liquid solution.

In normal individuals, most of the direct bilirubin first passes from the liver into the intestinal tract through the bile ducts, gallbladder, and common duct. From the intestines, direct bilirubin is eliminated in the stool, except for a small portion that is reabsorbed into the bloodstream. Since it has already been processed by the liver into a water-soluble form, any direct bilirubin returned to the circulation can now be readily eliminated by the kidneys into the urine.

Thus at any one time your blood contains some of the solubilized direct bilirubin as well as the unprocessed waste product of red blood cells, indirect bilirubin. Both kinds of bilirubin are measured as total bilirubin. This test has become routine.

In case of elevated bilirubin, your physician will order further tests to find out how much of each bilirubin there is, and whether one or both are responsible for the elevation. Of the maximum level of 1.2 milligrams of total bilirubin normally found in healthy individuals, the amount of direct bilirubin does not usually exceed 0.4 milligram, leaving a maximum of 0.8 milligram for indirect bilirubin.

An abnormal level of indirect bilirubin *only* indicates that the body's red blood cells may be breaking down at an excessive rate, as happens in hemolytic anemia. Excessive red blood cell destruction occurs because of exposure to certain industrial poisons and insecticides or as a side effect of some medications. Even though working normally, the liver may not be able to process the abnormal load of indirect bilirubin. Result? An abnormal buildup of indirect bilirubin in the blood.

An excessive buildup of indirect bilirubin may occur even when red blood cells are dying off at a normal rate. The cause of the problem this time? Indirect bilirubin literally backing up into the bloodstream because the liver cannot do its job. Indirect bilirubin may be unable to enter the liver in the first place because of swelling of liver tissues or some form of blockage. Or the liver may lack the necessary enzymes to convert indirect bilirubin into direct bilirubin.

Another possibility is that the conversion into direct bilirubin has been accomplished, but because of gallstones, tumors, infection, inflammation, or other problems involving the bile drainage system, the direct bilirubin cannot pass into the intestine. Instead of being eliminated in the feces, it is reabsorbed into the blood.

If the problem involves the bile drainage system or the liver, the direct bilirubin is likely to become more significantly elevated than the indirect bilirubin. The total may rise to 15 to 20 milligrams per 100 milliliters of serum. The physician will need to use other diagnostic tools to determine whether it is the bile drainage system or the liver that is primarily responsible for the elevation.

One clue may be the color of the stool. Patients with bile-duct disorders are likely to have bowel movements that become so light in color as to resemble clay. This is because the reddish bilirubin is unable to enter the intestinal tract. In liver problems, stools may be only slightly abnormal in color because bilirubin is still able to drain into the intestines.

Liver damage can occur in many situations, such as poisoning by certain chemicals, side effects from a number of common prescription drugs, and in such diseases as cirrhosis and hepatitis.

You may have known someone who developed a liver condition such as infectious hepatitis. Perhaps you noticed a yellowish color to his or her skin and even to the whites of the eyes. That is jaundice, which becomes evident when the total bilirubin exceeds 2.5 milligrams. The coloration is caused by the same bilirubin which imparts the deep brown color to normal feces. An alert laboratory technician may notice the jaundiced color of the blood even while preparing the serum sample for analysis. Extra precautions must be taken to avoid contact with such serum samples due to the possibility of viral hepatitis transmission.

You should not, however, mistake a similar yellowing sometimes seen in individuals interested in health foods and who consume large quantities of carrots or other yellow vegetables. The carotene pigments in such foods can discolor the blood serum and even color the skin, fingertips, and earlobes. The only indication that it is not jaundice: the whites of the eyes remain unaffected. Pediatricians are aware of this problem, which is quite common when an infant takes a liking to carrots and is given increasing amounts to indulge its preference for them. There is also a folk myth that eating lots of carrots will improve one's eyesight since carotene is essential for night vision. The attempt to obtain better vision by munching on carrots does not benefit most persons except to impart an orange hue to the skin which may be mistaken for a healthy glow or suntan.

---

*Blood constituent: Total Cholesterol*
Normal range: 140 to 265 milligrams per 100 milliliters (mg/100 ml)

---

Cholesterol today is a household word. Ever since a number of clinical studies in the late 1950s linked high levels of cholesterol with heart disease, cholesterol has received unprecedented publicity in the media. It has been singled out as the number-one dietary enemy of our health. The advertising community has felt free to use cholesterol as a sort of scapegoat to promote the sale of certain foods at the expense of others. Even children know that cholesterol is a dangerous thing lurking in our favorite foods.

The truth, in fact, is far more complex. Not only is the link between cholesterol and heart disease not as firm as it was once thought to be, but cholesterol in certain amounts is essential to life.

Cholesterol is the basis for synthesis of compounds that regulate some of the most important bodily processes. It makes possible the passage of vital substances through cell walls. It keeps us from becoming waterlogged when we bathe and spares us from becoming salt-depleted in hot climates. Cholesterol is even essential for the sex hormones which are involved in the sex drive and reproduction.

Cholesterol is closely related to various sex hormones in the body and to vitamin D. It is a fatty substance that, in pure form, looks like wax. One of the most important things to keep in mind about cholesterol is that the body can and does manufacture its own supply, regardless of what is found in the diet.

Over 70 percent of the total cholesterol in the blood is made in the liver, skin, adrenal glands, intestines, and testes or ovaries—with the liver accounting for the greater portion of this cholesterol production. Excess amounts tend to deposit in the walls of major blood vessels, impeding the flow of blood.

Most people have an ample intake of dietary cholesterol. It is in many of our basic foods: in meats, especially in fatty cuts; in dairy products; and in egg yolks. The highest concentration of cholesterol is in calves' brains—a delicacy in many French restaurants—closely followed by egg yolks.

Yet the link between how much cholesterol we eat and how much there is in our blood is not always in direct proportion. Granted, a diet lower in cholesterol will often result in slightly lowered cholesterol in the blood. Yet most healthy individuals can enjoy a diet relatively high in cholesterol with no appreciable change in the cholesterol levels.

On the other end of the scale are individuals who may have virtually cholesterol-free diets, yet are unable to lower appreciably the high levels of cholesterol in their blood. Some studies indicate that other constituents in the diet, such as high levels of sugar, may determine whether cholesterol in what we eat will be retained as excess cholesterol in the blood.

A further complication concerns the link between elevated levels of cholesterol and heart attacks. This link has not always been very clear. Why do some people with elevated levels of cholesterol remain well, while others become victims of heart attacks?

Persons who have cholesterol levels in excess of 300 milligrams per 100 milliliters are three times more susceptible to coronary heart disease than those with normal levels. Individuals who have cholesterol levels below 150 milligrams per 100 milliliters usually have no hazard of major heart disease. However, about 75 percent of all heart attacks occur in patients with cholesterol values in the normal range.

Why is this so?

Part of the answer appears to be in the way cholesterol combines with proteins and is transported in the blood. One type of combination is thought to be good for you and the other to be bad. The good cholesterol is found attached to high-density lipoprotein, or HDL; the bad cholesterol is associated with low-density lipoprotein, or LDL. Remember: in the case of HDL, high is good, low is bad.

Doctors are increasingly ordering the HDL test for patients who have anything more than very low levels of cholesterol. Here, the link seems to be far clearer. If you have a high proportion of HDL associated with the cholesterol, you have a far smaller chance of having a heart attack than if you have a high proportion of LDL, with its cholesterol. It is the LDL fraction of cholesterol which is thought to deposit plaque in your arteries and clog them up—like scale deposits in old water pipes. This is the process which frequently leads to atherosclerosis and heart attacks.

Within the normal range for cholesterol, if a male patient has an HDL level of about 45 milligrams per 100 milliliters, his heart disease risk factor is equal to the average of our population. For females, an average risk means about 55 milligrams of HDL. If the HDL level drops to about 30 milligrams, then the risk of coronary heart disease increases to double the average rate.

To reduce the risk of heart and blood vessel disease, it appears that you should strive to increase the relative amount of HDL in your blood. For people who have HDL levels in excess of 70 milligrams per 100 milliliters, the risk factor decreases to only half that for the general population.

One way to elevate your HDL level is, apparently, through physical exercise. Joggers and physically active people usually register an elevated HDL and decreased LDL in relation to their total cholesterol. Needless to say, HDL to LDL ratio is not the only risk factor in coronary heart disease. Other factors, such as your weight, amount of stress, smoking habits, blood pressure, and the overall health history of members of your family tree, are also contributory.

Women often register higher total cholesterol levels during pregnancy or while taking oral contraceptive pills. A saving grace is that the extra cholesterol is usually the HDL kind, which is caused by increased levels of estrogens formed during pregnancy or contained within the birth control pills. The practical problem in prescribing estrogens to raise HDL levels in order to reduce the chance of heart attacks is that estrogens have unacceptable side effects in both men and women.

Increases in cholesterol can be seen during the course of certain liver diseases, such as biliary cirrhosis or bile duct blockage, as well as in hypothyroidism, Cushing's syndrome, and, most common of all, uncontrolled sugar diabetes. Diabetic patients who have hardening of the arteries have higher cholesterol levels than diabetics without this complication. The question as to which comes first—the high cholesterol or the hardening of the arteries—has not yet been fully resolved.

As old age creeps up, the normal range for total cholesterol also increases. It is not uncommon for people over the age of sixty-five to have cholesterol values ranging up to 320 milligrams. But this "normality" confers no special protection; older people also are normally subject to higher rates of heart attacks.

There is much more to be learned about cholesterol. In the meantime, it would seem that the best way to play it safe would be to maintain a reasonable level of total cholesterol, with a high proportion of the good, HDL kind and as low a proportion as possible of the bad, LDL kind. And it seems to be well within our power to do so, provided we have the will to regulate our appetite for certain foods, even lobster, and to get adequate regular exercise. Even if we do not completely escape our genetic heritage, we can probably improve our health and our chances for longer survival.

---

*Blood constituent: Triglycerides*
Normal range: 50 to 170 milligrams per 100 milliliters (mg/100 ml)

---

As an indicator of potential heart disease, the simple test for fasting triglycerides was around for quite some time before testing for HDL cholesterol was developed. Today, most of the emphasis is on cholesterol and only rarely do you hear much about triglycerides. However, some physicians still regard the triglyceride test as a better indicator of possible heart trouble than cholesterol.

What are triglycerides? Look around, and you will probably see them in ample quantities in your immediate proximity, perhaps even on your own person. Triglycerides make up that midriff bulge, those heavy jowls, those fatty deposits in the thighs and buttocks. They are all concentrations of triglycerides, stored in special cells called adipose tissue. Triglycerides, in other words, are fat.

Where do triglycerides come from? To be sure, some of them come from our diet: meats, vegetable oils, butter, and other obvious sources. But triglycerides also are manufactured in the body, mainly in the liver. In fact, the liver is a major source of the triglycerides in your blood. Triglycerides in the liver are made from excess carbohydrates, especially from sugar and alcohol. One of the richest sources of triglycerides, therefore, would be that second milkshake, extra rich and extra sweet, fortified with eggnog mixture at holiday time.

Triglycerides certainly are not all bad. In limited amounts, triglycerides are essential to life. They are an important source of energy for your body. If you happened to be undergoing an enforced fast, triglycerides in the adipose tissues could serve as a major source of energy. These triglycerides have the highest caloric value per unit weight of any body material. Under fasting conditions, they are capable of providing up to 90 percent of your energy needs.

Of course, as the person uses up the triglycerides stored in adipose tissue, he or she will lose weight. The rate at which this stored fat can be released is often influenced by various hormones, as well as by caffeine and nicotine. That is why there may be some truth to the claim often made by smokers that whenever they try to stop smoking they gain weight.

The real culprits are not the deposits of triglycerides in the adipose tissues which present a cosmetic problem, but the triglycerides in the bloodstream. Shortly after triglycerides from what you eat enter the bloodstream, they form what are known as chylomicrons. Chylomicrons are microscopic droplets of triglycerides on their way to tissues for use in energy production or to adipose tissue for storage.

Chylomicrons persist in the bloodstream for about ten to twelve hours after eating before they reach their destinations. That is why, if you are being tested for excess triglycerides, you should refrain from eating for at least twelve hours. A non-fasting blood specimen could mistakenly show elevated results because it would also measure the triglycerides from the last meal.

Any inability of the body to remove these chylomicrons from the blood would cause elevated triglycerides. Other causes could include the excess intake of fats, sugars, or alcohol in the diet or the overproduction of triglycerides by the liver.

Why are triglycerides believed to be conducive to cardiovascular disease? You could perhaps judge for yourself if you had a chance to see a blood specimen with triglycerides of 300 or 400 milligrams per 100 milliliters, or even higher. The profusion of chylomicrons in such a specimen would turn it cloudy or even milky white. These globules of fatty materials in the blood can eventually deposit in the walls of arteries. Before this stage, they slow the normal blood circulation and increase the risk of heart attacks and other cardiovascular diseases.

The individual with elevated triglycerides, who may also have elevated cholesterol, can be treated with special fat-restricted diets containing little or no sugar and practically no alcohol. Sometimes, the physician may prescribe drug therapy along with the restrictive diet if symptoms of circulatory disorders are present. Exercise is usually helpful in reducing triglycerides.

Not all causes of elevated triglycerides will respond to diet. Yes, there are thin people with high triglycerides! Some of the problems may be related to genetic inheritance; the more resistant cases, to conditions such as severe deficiency of thyroid hormones. However, diet and exercise will usually help to some extent.

These recommendations may present a challenge if you have high triglycerides. But you should keep in mind that the lower the level of triglycerides in your blood, the lower the chances of developing complications in the circulatory system.

---

*Blood constituent: Total Protein*
Normal range: 6.0 to 8.5 grams per 100 milliliters (g/100 ml)

Protein is the major solid constituent dissolved in the liquid portion of your blood. Most other constituents are measured in milligrams; protein is measured in grams. In relative terms, there is a lot of it in your blood. The total proteins circulating in your blood can provide insights into your body's metabolic functions, the blood's capability of transporting nutrients to various parts of the body, and the defensive capability of your body.

The proteins in your blood are not in the same form as those you eat. The proteins from your diet are first digested into amino acids, which are the building blocks that make up proteins. The amino acids are then absorbed into your bloodstream through the upper intestine and carried to every tissue in your body. There are some twenty different amino acids, each distinct and separate. The tissues select whichever of these amino acids they may need to build the specific proteins necessary to fulfill their functions.

Among such protein-building tissues is your liver. The liver is where the proteins found in your blood are primarily formed. Once released by the liver into the bloodstream, the high-protein solution comes in contact with all of the body's cells and helps to preserve the fluid balance between cells and other body fluids.

As a general group of blood constituents, proteins are composed of several distinct types, each with its own specialized functions.

Albumin forms the largest share of these proteins in your blood, accounting for about 60 percent of their total in circulation. The remaining 40 percent are classified as globulins. Some of the globulins are formed in tissues other than the liver and provide specific immunity against disease.

Measurement of total proteins may not always be as revealing as testing specifically for albumin and the various globulins. But total protein does provide some useful indicators.

Total protein level in the blood will decrease if there is excessive protein elimination through the kidneys or if there is a chronic loss of blood from the body. Insufficient dietary protein intake or actual starvation can lead to decreased total protein concentration. The body will simply not have enough amino acids from which to build the proteins it may need. Advanced stages of hypertension when heart failure has developed, Hodgkin's disease of the lymph gland system, and certain types of leukemia may also reduce total protein levels. And, if excess fluid is temporarily retained in the body, the total concentration of proteins may be decreased because of the dilution effect.

The only common elevation of total protein is during dehydration due to the concentrating effect of the fluid loss. In both cases, the absolute supply of proteins in the body has not changed and no medical significance should be attached to such fluctuations. On the other hand, an unexplained high protein level may be an indicator of a major disorder such as multiple myeloma, an overproduction of proteins by tumorlike multiplication of plasma cells.

A note of interest: When the test for total proteins is made in the laboratory, the result does not include the weight of fibrinogen, also a protein. This is because the analysis is usually performed on serum rather than plasma. Since the clear serum is obtained from clotted blood, the amount of fibrinogen protein remaining in the serum is essentially zero, and the fibrinogen used up in the formation of the clot is discarded in the preparation of the sample.

---

*Blood constituent: Albumin*
Normal range: 3.5 to 5.5 grams per 100 milliliters (g/100 ml)

---

Of all the proteins circulating in your blood, albumin is the major constituent. It is a relatively small molecule, manufactured in your liver and ultimately returning to the liver to be broken down into its amino acid building blocks—only to start the cycle all over again.

Because of its small size, albumin plays a key role in maintaining the proper pressure between the fluids of your vascular system and the surrounding cells. In cases of spillover from one into the other, albumin can act as a sponge to absorb the fluid that has been filtered out and return it to its proper place. In other words, albumin helps keep the liquid portion of your blood from seeping out of your veins to form edema fluid.

Albumin also plays an important role in transporting chemicals, especially medications which do not readily dissolve in water, throughout your bloodstream. Typically, insoluble materials such as barbiturates, bilirubin, fatty acids, and various hormones are found attached to albumin. These insoluble materials would not be readily available for use by the needy tissues if albumin did not play its role in binding and transporting them to the appropriate locations within your body.

Because albumin represents a large proportion of all proteins, it is measured in routine screening profiles so as to provide more information about any changes in total proteins. It is common for the changes in the amount of albumin to parallel those of other proteins.

Malnutrition or starvation will provide a lower amount of protein to the body from which to obtain the necessary amino acids. Therefore, the albumin concentration may become reduced under these conditions.

Decreased albumin levels are also seen in some patients with kidney diseases which allow the small albumin molecule to escape through the kidney's filtration cells into the urine.

Decreased levels of albumin are often found in individuals with cirrhosis of the liver, infections, trauma, renal failure, and some gastrointestinal diseases. If the liver is damaged because of a disease condition such as hepatitis, the ability of the liver to produce albumin will be impaired, resulting in decreased levels of albumin.

The lowered concentration of albumin in the presence of severe illness may be a result of the body's increased need for amino acids elsewhere—and hence the inability of the liver to produce albumin due to a shortage of the basic materials for manufacturing it. The lowered albumin level will then be a secondary effect of a more specific problem elsewhere in the body.

Increased concentrations of albumin are not expected except when the body is dehydrated.

---

*Blood constituent: Globulins*
Normal range: 2.0 to 3.5 grams per 100 milliliters (g/100 ml)

---

Globulins are a class of proteins which include a wide variety of constituents. Globulins are basically transportation agents for many vital nutrients and other components in your blood. Some of the globulins also act as defense agents in various parts of your body.

The customary way to determine globulin levels in blood is to first measure the amounts of total protein and of albumin. The mathematical difference obtained by subtracting the albumin value from the total protein gives us the level of globulins.

Globulins themselves are made up of numerous subclasses and fractions. In patients with globulin levels above normal range, the physician will order a further breakdown in which the globulin proteins are identified by means of electrophoresis—separation in an apparatus with a high-voltage electrical field. This process reveals which of the globulins may be causing the problem.

Such a breakdown yields the various alpha and beta globulins, which serve as the moving vans of the bloodstream. Among their clients are such blood travelers as the sex hormones; hormones released by the thyroid gland; various forms of copper, iron, and cholesterol; as well as other bloodstream constituents of similar importance. For example, the beta globulin transferrin is involved in the metabolism of iron, so essential to formation of hemoglobin and your supply of oxygen. Without such globulins, iron and other vital constituents of the bloodstream simply would not be able to reach the places where they are most needed.

Of all the globulin fractions, gamma globulins are probably the best known. You have doubtless heard of people who experienced the discomfort of injections of gamma globulin after they had been exposed to a case of infectious hepatitis.

Gamma globulins are composed of a variety of protective antibodies. For example, during pregnancy the unborn fetus receives a supply of the mother's gamma globulin, which continues to safeguard the newborn until the baby can begin to make its own antibodies. If the newborn is susceptible to frequent infections, chances are that the child did not receive adequate gamma globulin protection from the mother or failed to start up its own assembly lines within its immune cell system.

Increased levels of gamma globulin may develop in individuals who suffer from allergies. These increased levels of gamma globulin are produced in response to foreign particles, like pollens that are inhaled by the lungs, or to foods that contain allergy-producing substances.

A general increase in gamma globulin fractions can also be seen as a response to many disease conditions such as infections, cirrhosis of the liver, various autoimmune diseases including hemolytic anemia, rheumatoid arthritis, a number of leukemias, lupus erythematosus, Hodgkin's disease, chronic liver diseases, and a widespread growth of microscopic plasma cells in organs and bones, known as multiple myeloma.

Decreases in gamma globulin may occur in kidney disease, agammaglobulinemia—which is the inability of the body to form sufficient antibodies—protein-losing diseases, chronic leukemia, lymphoma, and starvation.

The rise in total protein level above the high end of normal is very likely to be caused by an increased globulin concentration. The albumin level is usually normal or only slightly decreased when the total globulins are elevated.

The most frequent causes of such elevations are infections or multiple myeloma, a disease in which extraordinary amounts of globulin may appear in the blood. This type of abnormality requires immediate detailed investigation with more complex electrophoresis testing to identify the chemical nature of these globulins.

---

*Blood constituent: SGOT*
Normal range: 10 to 40 milliUnits per milliliter (mU/ml)

---

SGOT is the abbreviation for serum glutamic-oxalacetic transaminase. It is an enzyme found in varying concentrations in many key organs of your body.

An enzyme is basically a catalyst that helps other chemicals in your body to do their work. The specific function of SGOT is to help break down the proteins you eat and give you energy. Because of its function, SGOT is present in those tissues where this sort of activity takes place: the heart, liver, kidney, brain, skeletal muscles, spleen, and lungs.

Abnormal elevation of SGOT in the blood means there could be a disease affecting one or more of these tissues which contain significant amounts of the enzyme. SGOT levels may be useful in determining exactly which organ has been damaged, depending on the location of symptoms and other tests such as the electrocardiogram.

The heart muscle contains the highest concentration of this enzyme. Levels of SGOT in people who have had recent heart attacks may be up to ten times the upper limit of normal. But for this elevation to occur, there must be some actual damage to the heart muscle. During angina attacks when tissue destruction does not occur, SGOT will remain normal.

SGOT levels will rise significantly in various liver conditions. This happens because this enzyme from the damaged liver cells will be spilled in increasing quantities into the bloodstream, as for example in viral hepatitis, chemical poisoning, infectious mononucleosis, cirrhosis, obstructive jaundice, and similar liver problems.

The progress of liver diseases can be monitored by watching for changes in SGOT levels and by means of other enzyme determinations such as SGPT and alkaline phosphatase levels and a special test known as 5-prime-nucleotidase. A continuing increase in SGOT means an accelerated destruction of liver cells; a decrease signals a reversal of the destructive process and improvement by the patient.

Decreased concentrations of SGOT are occasionally seen during pregnancy because the enzyme is diluted by the increased buildup of fluids in the blood.

---

*Blood constituent:* SGPT
Normal range: 3 to 23 milliUnits per milliliter (mU/ml)

---

SGPT is another tongue-twister: serum glutamic-pyruvic transaminase. SGPT is an enzyme important in protein metabolism, which takes place primarily within the liver.

Analysis of SGPT is used specifically to determine the presence of liver cell damage. In case other enzyme elevations—such as LDH or SGOT—are detected, SGPT is used to find out whether the liver may or may *not* be responsible for the other abnormal enzyme levels. Any appreciable increase of SGPT in your blood confirms the likelihood that the liver is involved in a disease syndrome.

The degree of elevation may indicate both the kind and severity of the liver disorder. In hepatitis, for example, the level of SGPT in the blood may skyrocket to thousands of units per milliliter. In cirrhosis, on the other hand, the elevation is usually limited to hundreds of units. This, of course, does not mean that one disease is any less severe than the other, but reflects the rate at which liver cells are subject to damage.

---

*Blood constituent:* LDH
Normal range: 100 to 225 microUnits per milliliter ($\mu$U/ml)

---

LDH, or lactic dehydrogenase, is an enzyme that converts lactic acid to pyruvic acid. By virtue of this chemical reaction, LDH plays an important role in sugar metabolism and in your body's production of energy, carbon dioxide, and water. LDH is present in most of your body's tissues, with the heart containing proportionately more of this enzyme than your kidneys, liver, and skeletal muscles.

Elevated levels of LDH are likely whenever tissues containing high concentrations of LDH have been damaged—enabling the enzyme to leak out into the bloodstream.

Heart attacks are usually accompanied by high LDH levels. Within the first twenty-four hours after damage to the heart muscle, blood samples will show elevated levels of the enzyme. This level may persist for more than a week following initial chest pains. If the heart is stressed by congestive failure or inflammations termed myocarditis, the LDH tests also tend to be elevated but do not reach such high levels as in heart attack.

Extremely high LDH activity is seen in certain disorders of the blood cells. The condition known as megaloblastic anemia that can result from vitamin $B_{12}$ or folic acid deficiency will give LDH values five to ten times the upper limit of normal. Other anemias and certain leukemias will also show high LDH levels.

Liver damage can produce elevated LDH readings. The elevation will usually not be as dramatic as with heart muscle damage, since the concentration of LDH in the liver is less than in the heart. Hepatitis, cirrhosis, or obstructive jaundice, for example, will cause a rise in LDH of two or three times the upper limit of the normal range for this test.

If the cause of elevated LDH in the blood is not readily evident, the physician may order further analysis of the LDH to pinpoint its origin. This can be done because LDH is an enzyme that is actually made up of five separate proteins. Each is associated with different specific tissues; one with your heart, another with your kidneys, another with your liver, and so forth. By finding out which one of the LDH factors is elevated, the site of disease can often be located.

Falsely elevated LDH readings may result from improper taking or handling of the blood specimen. Any destruction of the red blood cells while the specimen is drawn or any rough treatment of the blood in the tube will cause LDH to be released from the cells into the serum. The analysis, then, will measure not only the normal presence of LDH in the specimen, but also the added amount of LDH from the red cell breakdown. The laboratory technician may note hemolysis, or a red-tinged appearance, that could account for the elevated LDH, and a replacement blood specimen will be requested.

---

*Blood constituent: Alkaline Phosphatase*
Normal range: 30 to 110 milliUnits per milliliter (mU/ml)

---

Alkaline phosphatase is an enzyme which is highly concentrated in your bones and liver, and to a lesser extent, in your spleen, kidneys, and intestines. Whenever there is damage to the bones or liver, this enzyme will usually leak out into the bloodstream in greater than normal amounts—and this serves as a good check on disorders of the major organ systems.

Abnormal amounts of alkaline phosphatase do not always mean you have a liver or bone disease. It could merely be a sign of unusual bone cell activity. Such increased activity is quite normal in youngsters, whose bones are still growing, and in people recovering from fractures. Alkaline phosphatase levels will also increase in a woman's blood during the last three months of pregnancy. This is because the placenta becomes an important source of the enzyme.

In bone disease, elevation of serum alkaline phosphatase is caused by such disorders as rickets, metastatic cancers from other tissues, or by parathyroid gland overactivity.

In liver disease, alkaline phosphatase is useful for determining the probable location and extent of the disease. The alkaline phosphatase in the liver is concentrated along the countless bile canals and ducts which are spread throughout the organ like a network of drainage pipes. Although any damage to this drainage system will cause an abnormal release of alkaline phosphatase into the blood, rather high levels are seen only when blockage of the major ducts is nearly complete. Slight changes in alkaline phosphatase levels may attract attention to the gallbladder as a site of possible disease, such as gallstones.

It is the degree of elevation which will help the doctor make a diagnosis—combined with other blood chemistry levels such as SGOT, SGPT, LDH, and bilirubin. In individuals with liver cancer, for example, alkaline phosphatase values may jump to twenty-five times the normal limit. Gallstones may increase the level up to ten times the upper limit of normal. Hepatitis, cirrhosis, and reactions to drugs usually have their own characteristic elevations which, again, can best be interpreted in conjunction with other lab findings and clinical observations.

---

*Blood constituent: Calcium*
Normal range: 8.5 to 10.5 milligrams per 100 milliliters (mg/100 ml)

---

Calcium plays a highly diversified role in the functioning of your body. By weight it is easily the most plentiful mineral in the body. Your bones and teeth store over 99 percent of this calcium; yet the remaining 1 percent, which is dissolved in your bloodstream, is essential to maintaining the strength of your bones, the contraction of your muscles, the proper transmission of nerve impulses, the clotting of your blood, and the activity of several enzymes vital to your body metabolism.

For most people in the United States, the major sources of calcium are milk and milk products, with such alternate sources as green leafy vegetables, legumes such as soybeans, eggs, meats, and, increasingly, various calcium supplements.

On the average, the amount of calcium your body absorbs each day from the diet is 125 milligrams. This just about equals the amount that is normally excreted in the urine each day. In active bone formation—during childhood, in pregnancy, or after a fracture—the amount of calcium in the urine is reduced because the body retains more to build new bone.

What happens is that the fresh calcium from your food replaces, in about equal amounts, the calcium that has been around in your body for some time. This replacement is part of a continuous process of rebuilding the crystalline structure of the skeleton. In essence, your bones are like coral reefs and your body fluids are like the sea, always building but always changing the structure.

Your body has two main reservoirs of calcium, your bloodstream and your bones. About half of the calcium in your blood is tied to albumin and other protein constituents. In this bound form, the calcium cannot penetrate the capillary walls and must remain in the blood as a reservoir. The other half is known as free calcium. It can readily pass through capillary walls and reach tissue cells to perform many necessary functions throughout your body.

When the laboratory measures calcium, it usually reports only the total level of calcium in your blood. But even with a normal level of calcium, the doctor may suspect a low effective calcium level if there are signs of bone disease or symptoms of calcium deficiency. If the albumin concentration is measured, an estimate can be made of the free calcium, which does the actual work. For even greater accuracy, there is a chemical test for free calcium which is done with a fresh sample of unclotted blood and special equipment.

Your body's largest reservoir of calcium is in the bones. There is a constant exchange between the free calcium from your bloodstream and the calcium deposits in your bones. The way your blood levels of calcium are kept normal is mainly through the right amount of give-and-take in this dynamic exchange.

The process is a very delicate one. The key to its success is a hormone produced by the parathyroid glands, hidden behind the thyroid gland in the front of your neck below the Adam's apple. The parathyroid hormone—known as PTH—is secreted whenever the level of free calcium in your blood falls below the minimum normal limit. The release of PTH has three immediate consequences:

1. PTH mobilizes free calcium from the bones, enabling this calcium to enter the bloodstream.

2. PTH enhances the return by the kidneys of calcium that would otherwise be excreted in the urine.

3. PTH stimulates the production of biologically active vitamin D, which is responsible for the absorption of calcium in the intestine.

If you have ever wondered why vitamin D is invariably added to milk, here is the answer: calcium metabolism. All that calcium in the milk you drink is of little use to your body unless there is enough vitamin D available—either in your body or in the milk. Vitamin D is not only essential for the proper absorption of calcium from the intestines, but it also helps in bone formation and in the action of PTH in releasing free calcium from your bones.

When the level of free calcium in the bloodstream reaches normal, it halts the secretion of PTH. With it, the three factors that were building up the levels of free calcium also come to a complete halt. If other factors cause the level of blood calcium to increase beyond normal, specialized "C" cells in the thyroid gland secrete a material called calcitonin which stops the release of free calcium from the bone. Calcitonin, in effect, acts as a counterbalance to the effects of PTH and vitamin D on bone—or to any other cause of very high serum free calcium.

You can see why abnormal levels of calcium could be due to a wide range of disorders. Too much calcium could result from improper functioning of the parathyroid glands—and could cause depletion of calcium from the bone. Intoxication with vitamin D can also cause this type of problem with serious consequences such as heart block or coma. Self-treatment with such supplements or well-intentioned overdosage of infants with this vitamin can be too much of a good thing and must be avoided.

High serum calcium, persistent levels of PTH, loss of bone density, and calcium stone formation in the urine are hallmarks of primary hyperparathyroidism. The usual cause is a single benign tumor of any one of the parathyroid glands. In some cases, all four of these glands become overactive and cause calcium loss from the bones until three glands or even all except a portion of one gland are surgically removed to reduce PTH secretion to normal. Removal of a tumor is dramatically curative after the dormant remaining glands revive in about five days after surgery. The bones tend to heal so rapidly that blood calcium may drop below normal, a situation familiarly known as "thirsty bones."

Too little serum calcium could signify a parathyroid gland deficiency, kidney disorder, intestinal absorption difficulties, or vitamin D deficiency.

A detailed understanding of how the calcium balance is maintained shows how intricate and complex the workings of your body really are. And as long as you are healthy, all this is done automatically and accurately without any sensation of the many events that are taking place throughout your body.

---

*Blood constituent: Phosphorus*
Normal range: 2.5 to 4.5 milligrams per 100 milliliters (mg/100 ml)

---

The major storage area for phosphorus is in the bones, which contain about 80 to 90 percent of the total phosphorus in the body. The rest is found in the body's soft tissues, which require phosphorus for such tasks as carbohydrate metabolism and muscle contraction. Phosphorus also plays an important part in the formation of genetic material and of such tissues as the brain and spinal cord.

The phosphorus in the bones unites with calcium to form an insoluble combination that gives the skeleton its shape and structural strength. A little-known function of the skeleton is that of providing a substantial reservoir of phosphorus, which has a neutralizing effect on acids when the blood becomes too acidic and exceeds tolerable limits.

Phosphorus is found in just about any food source—whether milk, meat, or leafy vegetables. It is easily absorbed from the gastrointestinal tract, and the body can readily put it to good use. The major path of elimination for phosphorus is similarly simple. About 60 percent goes out in the urine, and the rest in the feces.

The level of phosphorus in your blood can vary with the time of day, your age, and the amount of time elapsed since your last meal. If the phosphorus concentration is measured too soon after a meal, the phosphorus level may read deceptively low. This is because the phosphorus will be busy helping to transport sugar molecules out of the bloodstream into the body's cells. While engaged in this task, phosphorus will temporarily lose its own identity and escape measurement.

Your body maintains a stable level of phosphorus in the blood through various means. If your phosphorus level falls below 3.2 milligrams and you are in normal health, then your kidneys will begin to reabsorb most of the phosphorus that was being excreted into your urine. Through this action, your phosphorus level will be stabilized, and may even begin to rise.

If your level is above 3.2 milligrams per 100 milliliters, the phosphorus lost in your urine will reflect the amount consumed in the diet.

The amount of phosphorus eliminated in the urine can be increased by activation of the parathyroid gland. Above-normal parathyroid hormone secretions will prevent the kidneys from reabsorbing the usual amounts of phosphorus in the filtration process. Hence, more phosphorus will be expelled and there will be a decrease in the phosphorus level in the bloodstream.

Vitamin D can have the opposite effect. It will raise the level of phosphorus in the blood by improving the ability of the kidneys to reabsorb phosphorus that would otherwise be excreted in the urine.

The proportions of calcium and phosphorus in your blood are very delicately balanced. As we have seen, the parathyroid hormone, vitamin D, and the ability of your kidneys to reabsorb phosphorus work together to stabilize the ratio of calcium to phosphorus in your blood.

If there is an increase in calcium concentration, an increase in the phosphorus level, or both, then an insoluble combination of the calcium and phosphorus will form and be deposited in certain tissues. This has been characterized as the "calcium X phosphorus product," which can force calcium to combine with phosphorus and form crystals.

What this means in practical terms is that when crystal formation takes place in the urine, it may create kidney stones. This could be especially true if your urine is alkaline—providing an ideal medium for the formation of calcium stones. Individuals with these types of stones have to reduce their intake of foods high in calcium.

A low level of phosphorus can mean that dietary intake or intestinal absorption of this substance is inadequate. One of the most common causes of low phosphorus is the frequent use of antacids, which bind phosphorus and cause it to be eliminated in the stool. If the low phosphorus is due to diarrhea, and calcium is also lost, the combined deficiency can cause bone formation to suffer.

There usually are no symptoms associated with low phosphorus. Screening tests are virtually the only way to identify this condition.

What can cause a high level of phosphorus in the blood? In the old days, it often used to be phosphorus poisoning from the matches of the type used to light pipe tobacco or fireplace kindling. This was a major hazard in the home; children chewed on them. Safety matches have eliminated that danger. Another potential hazard is the various phosphate fertilizers so essential to growing our farm produce. But these are easily removed with washing and have not presented any measurable phosphorus poisoning so far.

Kidney poisoning is actually the main cause of high phosphorus levels in the blood. A major sign of such kidney failure is the rise of phosphorus above normal limits in the blood. Since the kidney is the sole check on phosphorus absorption, this process will then continue unchecked by any other internal protective system.

High phosphorus can be treated by taking advantage of the same process that causes low phosphate; i.e., using antacids to bind the phosphorus before it can be absorbed. But this treatment may not be utilized until kidney function improves or dialysis treatment is started, since a certain level of kidney function is essential for sustaining life.

---

*Blood constituent: Sodium*
Normal range: 135 to 147 milliEquivalents per liter (mEq/L)

---

The basic purpose of this test is to determine any salt or electrolyte imbalance in your body. An imbalance could be related to possible kidney or adrenal-gland disorders.

To understand electrolyte imbalance, we'll have to backtrack for a moment. There are four main electrolytes in your bloodstream. In addition to sodium, these are chloride, potassium, and carbon dioxide in the form of bicarbonate. Sodium and potassium are positively charged ions. Chloride and carbon dioxide as bicarbonate are negatively charged ions. At any moment in your body, the number of positively charged ions has to equal those carrying a negative charge. That is why electrolytes are measured in milliEquivalents, which indicate the number of electrical charges per liter of fluid. It is the number of these charges rather than the actual weight that is the key factor in the regulation of salt distribution needed to achieve a perfect balance throughout your body fluids.

Of all the salts in your body, sodium is the most plentiful. It is found just about everywhere: in the blood; within the internal organ tissues; in muscles and bones; in the brain and its cerebrospinal fluid; in nerves, tears, sweat, gastric juices, and urine.

Sodium is best known as the main component of common table salt, the other component being chloride. But sodium is also contained in most foods in sufficient quantities to satisfy the normal needs of your body. Whatever salt you happen to sprinkle on your food is usually eliminated by the kidneys into your urine. It is estimated that most people use about ten times as much salt as their body actually needs to replace that which is lost in the sweat, urine, or stools under normal conditions.

Sodium serves many vital purposes in your body. These range from helping to carry nutrients and wastes to and from cells, to transmitting electrical impulses throughout your nervous system, to giving you control over your voluntary bodily movements, to supporting the automatic functions of the intestinal tract.

Sodium has a key role in maintaining the proper water volume and pressure in body tissues. The tone and shape of the cells are in part the result of the amount of water in each cell. Sodium prevents water from overloading the cells by keeping the water in the bloodstream and in the fluids which bathe the body cells.

In effect, sodium acts like a sponge. Wherever sodium goes, water must follow to preserve the normal salt concentration. If sodium is increased, then the water volume tends to increase.

The result is an increased volume of blood and hence a possible increase in blood pressure. That is the reason why low-salt diets are generally prescribed for patients with high blood pressure. Another result is an increase in the volume of water surrounding the body's cells outside the bloodstream. Known as edema, this condition is marked by swelling around the ankles and other parts of the body. Edema is sometimes coupled with high blood pressure and requires the same low-salt regimen.

When sodium intake is restricted, there is a reduction of water in the bloodstream and in the body's cells. This results in lowered blood pressure and loss of weight, in the form of water passed as urine. That is why most weight-reducing diets counsel a reduction of salt intake. However encouraging the weight loss may prove, it does not represent a true reduction in fatty tissue.

How does the body maintain the delicate balance of just the right amount of sodium—especially when you consider the large intake of salt by the majority of our population?

The kidneys and the adjacent adrenal glands are responsible for this task. It is the job of the kidneys, after filtering the urine, to reabsorb the proper amount of sodium. If the diet is low in salt, then the body compensates by reabsorbing more sodium. The adrenal glands release a hormone called aldosterone which stimulates the kidneys to perform the needed increased absorption of sodium. At the same time, water is reabsorbed with the salt as a secondary effect, and the fluid volume of the blood is restored to normal.

A high sodium level in the body may indicate that an adrenal gland tumor has developed and is releasing too much aldosterone in an unregulated pattern. This condition is known as primary aldosteronism.

High sodium levels can also be caused when you do not drink enough water to replace what you normally lose through urine and perspiration. This state of dehydration can happen more readily to sick or very elderly persons who may not be able to care for themselves properly. It is for this reason that hospital patients are monitored with a continuous listing of all fluids taken in and the total volume of urine produced each day.

A deficiency in antidiuretic hormone can result in increased sodium levels because the kidneys are unable to reabsorb the necessary amounts of filtered water. Marked by frequent urination and extreme thirst, this condition is known as diabetes insipidus. As the name implies, the urine is insipid, or tasteless, and resembles pure tap water in appearance.

Low blood levels of sodium can result if the kidneys cannot reabsorb enough sodium. This problem can be caused by the inability of the adrenal glands to secrete sufficient quantities of aldosterone because of damage to either the adrenal glands or the kidneys. Or the kidneys may be unable to eliminate the necessary amount of water, the backup diluting the sodium present in the body. Such conditions as cirrhosis of the liver, congestive heart failure, Addison's disease, severe diabetes, and hypothyroidism are often accompanied by decreased blood sodium levels. Decreased sodium may also be caused by such relatively common conditions as excessive sweating or diarrhea, and by the use of diuretic drugs.

Significantly high or low sodium levels can lead to severe problems in the functioning of the nervous system. In essence, sodium and other salts act similarly to electrolytes in a storage battery. They provide the chemical environment which allows energy to flow in the form of charged ions or molecules. Just as a battery must have the proper amount of water and acid to function at top performance, no less does your body require balanced conditions with respect to sodium and water content.

---

*Blood constituent: Chloride*
Normal range: 95 to 110 milliEquivalents per liter (mEq/L)

---

As with sodium, the purpose of the chloride test is to detect any electrolyte imbalance. Most of the information applicable to sodium is valid for chloride.

Chloride is the companion component to sodium in ordinary table salt. Chloride is also present in many of the foods we eat.

In your body, chloride is found in the same tissues and fluids as sodium and potassium. The highest concentration is in gastric juice in the form of hydrochloric acid.

With chloride ions having a single negative charge and sodium and potassium ions each having a positive charge, the body remains in a state of electrical neutrality. Although there are other positively and negatively charged particles in the body, sodium and chloride are by far the most numerous. That is why when the two salts are present in their proper proportions, the body's electrical neutrality is assured.

Your body maintains its chloride balance through virtually the same mechanism as its sodium balance. Chloride migrates passively with sodium or potassium as a pair of ions and is reabsorbed or excreted in comparable quantities.

Lower than normal chloride may be the result of excessive sweating, diarrhea, or vomiting. Reduced chloride levels could also be a sign of more serious conditions such as the adrenal gland deficiency known as Addison's disease, intestinal obstruction, or a condition known as metabolic acidosis, usually found in diabetic conditions.

Abnormally high levels of chloride in the blood can be a result of water loss without adequate replacement, such as in untreated diabetes insipidus. Other causes could be excessive use of ammonium chloride expectorants and overbreathing, or hyperventilation. What happens in hyperventilation is that a negative chloride ion is retained as a replacement for a negative bicarbonate ion that is lost through the excessive breathing.

Together with sodium, potassium, and bicarbonate levels, the measurement of chloride provides important clues to the state of salt or electrolyte balance within the body. All four are frequently measured in the monitoring of postoperative patients, especially after intestinal surgery or other situations in which intravenous fluids are the major or only source of nutrients and minerals.

*Blood constituent: Potassium*
Normal range: 3.5 to 5.5 milliEquivalents per liter (mEq/L)

Potassium is the major mineral constituent found inside your body's cells. Potassium is essential for muscle contraction and is involved in many of the metabolic processes of starch and sugar.

The normal level of this vital mineral in your cells is maintained by the potassium contained in your diet. Bananas and oranges are especially high in potassium. The average diet has sufficient potassium, 60 to 80 milliEquivalents, to meet or exceed the body's daily needs.

The potassium in your diet is used primarily to replace the potassium lost through the urine. The kidneys do not have the ability to reabsorb potassium being excreted, and this normal loss must be replenished from the diet. A lesser amount of potassium is lost in sweat and in the stool. Some potassium may be needed when new tissue is formed after injuries or healing of burns.

Because of potassium's role in the proper contraction of your muscles, it is essential to maintain an adequate concentration of this mineral in your body fluids. Nerve fibers are also rich in potassium, using it as a conductor for nerve impulses.

Potassium thus enables you to make the body do what you want it to do. Without enough potassium, you might experience muscular weakness, cramps, and a general lethargy. Should low potassium levels continue over extended periods, the result could be partial paralysis of the hands and legs and interference with the heartbeat.

Potassium is vital to the heart. Without enough potassium, your heart would not contract—and might, in fact, stop beating. On the other hand, too much potassium could also cause severe disturbances of the heart. If the potassium level should reach 10 milliEquivalents per liter, your heart muscle would stop contracting altogether.

The body's regulation of blood potassium is not very precise. If elevations occur above the high end of the normal range, then more of the hormone aldosterone will be released from the adrenal glands to cause increased elimination of potassium through the kidneys.

Low levels of blood potassium have to be replenished by diet or supplements. Patients who are receiving diuretic medications for high blood pressure are usually watchful of their potassium levels. They may need extra potassium-rich foods in their diet or potassium supplements.

In measuring elevated potassium levels, care must be taken to interpret the results properly. Any damage to the red blood cells prior to analysis—through heat or undue delay—may result in the release of potassium from the blood cells into the serum. This would produce erroneously elevated results. Likewise, the tiny clot-promoting elements in the blood known as platelets may release potassium if the specimen is left to stand. This is especially likely when these particles are present in high numbers, as in the blood disorder known as polycythemia vera. Mistaken higher readings could prove dangerous for patients whose potassium levels might, in fact, be less than adequate and in need of treatment. If the laboratory report includes the brief notation "hemolysis," the physician becomes wary of the result and orders another sample.

Another means of monitoring the potassium result is to examine the electrocardiogram. Your physician can recognize signs of low body potassium by the appearance of low T waves—a bump in the recording that follows each electrical contraction spike. The opposite situation can also be seen—very high, "peaked" T waves—when body potassium is above normal. Since many factors can influence this electrical pattern, laboratory confirmation of a change in potassium is needed, but both tests complement each other.

---

*Blood constituent: Carbon Dioxide as Bicarbonate*
Normal range: 20 to 30 milliEquivalents per liter (mEq/L)

---

As you use up the oxygen you inhale, carbon dioxide is released by your body cells. But before the carbon dioxide can bubble off as gas, it is converted in your blood to bicarbonate by the action of red blood cells.

Bicarbonate is no mystery compound. It is identical to the all-purpose baking soda on your pantry shelf.

Most of the bicarbonate dissolved in your blood is carried to your lungs. It is mainly here that the bicarbonate is finally eliminated as carbon dioxide, in exchange for a new supply of oxygen.

Like chloride, bicarbonate is a negatively charged ion. Together these two salts make up the bulk of negatively charged particles in your blood. They are responsible for maintaining a balance with the positively charged particles, comprised primarily of sodium, potassium, and calcium.

The lungs as well as the kidneys are involved in controlling the bicarbonate level in your blood. If you hyperventilate—that is, breathe too rapidly—you will lose too much carbon dioxide and develop a low bicarbonate level in your blood. This condition is called respiratory alkalosis and is marked by spasms of the hand and foot muscles and a sense of impending suffocation. Other causes of low bicarbonate are hysteria, anxiety, fever, increased ketones from starvation or diabetes, diarrhea, and kidney or central nervous system diseases.

High levels of bicarbonate in the blood can result from hypoventilation or inadequate exchange of air. Hypoventilation can be caused by fluid in the lungs or by drug poisoning that affects the breathing control center in the brain, which responds to the level of carbon dioxide in the blood. Increased bicarbonate in the blood is called respiratory acidosis. It can produce coma and even death.

Special care must be taken in handling the blood sample before analysis. Since, in the presence of oxygen, bicarbonate can readily break down into carbon dioxide and escape, the sample should never be exposed to air. This is best assured by drawing a full tube of blood and eliminating any possible air space. The purpose of the test is defeated if this procedure is not carried out as described.

---

*Blood constituent: Iron*
Normal range: 50 to 180 micrograms per 100 milliliters (mcg or
    $\mu$g/100 ml)

---

In most organisms, iron is an essential element for sustaining life. Yet the quantities present in your bloodstream are minuscule, measured in micrograms rather than the usual milligrams for most other vital materials.

Iron is the active component of hemoglobin, the oxygen-carrying portion of the red blood cells. Over 70 percent of the body's iron is incorporated into hemoglobin. Most of the balance of the iron is in storage in the serum portion of the blood, in the liver, and in the bone marrow.

The daily consumption of iron in the diet varies between 5 and 15 milligrams. In a normal state, however, the body absorbs only about one-tenth of this amount; so most of the iron must be recycled. The amount of iron your body actually uses from the diet—from 0.5 to 2.0 milligrams—approximates the amount of iron that is normally lost every day. Such loss usually occurs through sweating, shedding of skin cells, and elimination in the urine and feces.

Absorption of iron from the diet will increase when the body is undergoing growth, pregnancy, or lactation, which create a greater demand for iron. The loss of iron during menstruation also requires increased uptake from the diet; however, an average balanced diet should provide a sufficient quantity of iron to meet even these increased demands.

What about all the iron needed to replace the iron in the hemoglobin of all those red blood cells that are constantly dying and being regenerated as part of the body's ongoing process of renewal?

The answer is that your body is able to recover iron in this form. When red blood cells break down, the iron from hemoglobin is redistributed to the various iron storage depots. This is done by means of a special protein, appropriately enough called transferrin. As iron is needed to produce fresh hemoglobin for new red blood cells, the iron in storage is released and again transported by transferrin; this time, to the active sites of manufacture of new red cells in the bone marrow.

In adult males and females, this cycle of storage, release, and resynthesis draws on the existing stores of body iron. In adult males, the body has sufficient reserves to meet such requirements for up to three years even if no iron is taken in from the diet. In females undergoing pregnancy, lactation, or normal menstruation, the iron reserves are not as extensive but still adequate.

If this is the case, then why are there such problems as iron deficiency anemia and low blood iron—in which iron supplements have to be taken?

The specific cause of individual problems has to be investigated by the physician, but here are several such possibilities: Decreased levels of serum iron can result from chronic blood loss in the intestinal tract due to hiatus hernia, an ulcer, or intestinal parasites; from decreased iron absorption over a period of time; or from a decreased intake of foods containing iron—especially in the case of females, since their requirements are greater. Excessive menstrual bleeding can place an extra burden on iron stores and result in anemia. This problem ceases after the change of life or after hysterectomy.

The levels of blood iron may also be reduced during some infections because of a failure to liberate enough iron from the hemoglobin of red blood cells undergoing normal breakdown. Moderate decreases in blood iron are common in chronic kidney diseases, rheumatoid arthritis, and cancer.

To help determine the probable reasons for decreased iron levels, the physician may also order an analysis of transferrin. The evaluation of this special protein is done by measuring its iron-binding capacity. If the binding capacity is high, this means that the condition is related to iron deficiency anemia. In other words, there is not enough iron around for the transferrin to transport to the key points within the body. If the binding capacity is low, then the problem could be that the transferrin is not doing its job and is causing the anemia. To further determine the cause of low binding capacity of transferrin could require a lot of medical sleuthing.

Among the most common reasons today for an elevated level of iron due to elevated transferrin are the oral contraceptive drugs. This does not mean that oral contraceptives can cure iron deficiency anemia or resolve a transferrin problem. They only increase the capacity to store iron in the bloodstream without providing more iron for the manufacture of new red blood cells.

Elevated levels of iron are also seen in certain pathological states such as lead poisoning, where there is an accelerated breakdown of red blood cells, a decreased formation of fresh red blood cells, and a defect in the ability of iron to combine with hemoglobin. If the liver is damaged, improper release of its stored iron will also cause elevated serum iron.

The average concentration of serum iron in normal adult males is 125 micrograms per 100 milliliters and 110 micrograms for females. As old age approaches, the average level for both sexes tends to decrease to about 70 micrograms. In newborn children, the level may exceed 200 micrograms, but this will gradually decrease to normal levels of 110 to 125 micrograms.

If the red cell count and hemoglobin determination are only border-line low, a low serum iron may provide a diagnosis. When hemorrhage from a peptic ulcer or from menstrual bleeding has been significant, tests for serum iron can establish the degree of deficiency and be used to follow up the results of taking iron pills.

# 6
# The Complete Blood Count

The complete blood count, or CBC, enables your physician to get a microscopic view of the two main cellular components of your blood, the red cells and the white cells. Together, they make up most of the blood's solid volume.

This close-up profile of your blood spares no details. It seeks to establish not only how many of these cells there are, but also such specifics as how big they are, what their oxygen-carrying capacity is, and how well they are able to fight off disease. This kind of test is routine in every clinical laboratory and is performed even in many doctors' offices.

Finding out such details about the billions of cells propelled along your bloodstream may be fascinating in itself. But the main purpose of the complete blood count is to uncover anything from potentially severe disease conditions—and how best to treat them—to perhaps discovering that your feeling of fatigue may really be no cause for concern after all.

In the adult, both red and white blood cells begin their development in the bone marrow contained within the flat bones of the skull, ribs, pelvis, spine, clavicle, and breastbone. In children and young adults, the long bones of the arms and legs also produce blood cells.

Whether red cells or white cells—erythrocytes or leukocytes—all cells have progressive stages of growth and development. In normal, healthy individuals the amount of mature red and white cells in the bloodstream remains fairly constant. Old cells die and are removed from the blood while new cells, created in the bone marrow, take their place.

The complete blood count seeks to determine whether this process is functioning smoothly. Any irregularities could be a response to subtle disease conditions which may be difficult to discover through any other tests or examinations.

---

*Total Red Blood Cell Count (RBC)*
Normal range, males: 4.2 to 5.4 million per cubic millimeter
Normal range, females: 3.6 to 5.0 million per cubic millimeter

---

The total red blood cell count is one of the most important of all laboratory tests.

It takes approximately six days for a red cell to develop in the bone marrow and be released into the blood. Shaped like a pancake with a central dimple, the mature red blood cell functions for 100 to 140 days. After that, it dies and is replaced. The red blood cells in the body, therefore, are replaced completely about three times each year.

The main purpose of your red cells is to transport oxygen from your lung tissues to support life throughout your body. Over 90 percent of the dry weight of each red blood cell consists of a substance called hemoglobin. Hemoglobin is the material in red blood cells which combines with oxygen from the air you breathe and carries it to its destinations.

An increased concentration of red cells beyond the normal range is called polycythemia. Polycythemia is not always a sign of some basic disorder. Sometimes the red cell count will become elevated when the total blood fluid volume is decreased because of diarrhea, vomiting, or other causes of dehydration. The total amount of red blood cells has remained normal, but their number per unit of liquid blood has increased because of reduced fluid volume.

Polycythemia may also be a normal response if you happen to reside at a high altitude. There the air is thinner and your body responds to lower oxygen availability by producing more oxygen-carrying red cells. Under such conditions of increased oxygen needs, a special hormone, erythropoietin, is released from the kidneys to stimulate the bone marrow to produce more cells.

This special hormone may be erroneously released when there is a tumor in one of the kidneys or in a related organ. Since no additional red cells are in fact needed, the resulting excess will thicken the blood and cause circulatory problems.

A similar condition, polycythemia vera, usually affects men over sixty. Their main laboratory finding is an increased concentration of red blood cells. These men usually have a ruddy facial appearance which conceals a major health problem. The origin of this chronic disease is unknown. Victims may make frequent blood donations, not so much to help others as to help themselves by removing the surplus blood, thus preventing high blood pressure or blood clot complications. Polycythemia vera probably inspired the old practice of bleeding the patient— no matter what the condition—especially in the case of older men. George Washington and others of his era were bled as a routine procedure to improve their health. Chances are, a number of them did actually suffer from polycythemia vera—and improved dramatically. In other cases, bleeding weakened already weak patients and undoubtedly hastened their deaths.

Still another form of red cell overproduction is known as secondary polycythemia. It generally afflicts people who have lung conditions such as emphysema or a form of congenital heart disease. Because their blood cannot properly draw on the oxygen in the lungs or supply such vital organs as the heart with adequate oxygen, their body tries to compensate by manufacturing more red blood cells. The mechanism at work is the same as what happens with healthy individuals at high altitudes. But the results are not similarly benign.

What if your problem is the opposite—not enough red blood cells? This condition, where the number of red blood cells falls below the normal range, is typical of many types of anemia. Marked by fatigue, breathlessness, and general malaise, anemia in its many forms is basically a red blood cell problem. It has been estimated that as many as 20 million people in the United States suffer from some form of anemia.

In one type of anemia, the decreased production of red cells can result when not enough of the bone-marrow-stimulating hormone is released by the kidneys due to kidney disease. Or it can be caused by cancers within the bone marrow, as in leukemia. In leukemia, the body undergoes a shift in its ability to manufacture red cells because of uncontrolled white cell overproduction.

Direct damage to the bone marrow tissue can also cause a decrease in the manufacture of red cells. When destruction of bone marrow tissue occurs, the condition is known as aplastic anemia. It is a debilitating disease which, if not checked, can often prove fatal.

Aplastic anemia is quickly becoming one of the severe diseases of our modern world. Although some of the causes of aplastic anemia are unknown, known causes include exposure to various commercially used chemicals such as the solvent benzene; some insecticides; and various anti-cancer drugs, as well as more common prescription drugs such as many tranquilizers, sulfonamides, and the antibiotics streptomycin and chloramphenicol. Many physicians will no longer prescribe chloramphenicol unless they are able to monitor the patient's red blood cell count and serum iron level at frequent intervals.

Anemia may also result from the increased destruction of the mature red blood cells to such a degree that the bone marrow is unable to replace them at the same rate. The bone marrow may be producing normally, but it just cannot keep up with the abnormal rate of destruction. This condition is known as hemolytic anemia.

Hemolytic anemia may be caused by environmental chemicals which can sharply decrease the life span of each cell. Or the body may actually produce antibodies against its own red cells, destroying them. This sometimes happens to individuals who have leukemia, certain types of malignant tumors, syphilis, infectious hepatitis, or the connective-tissue disease known as lupus erythematosus.

Hemolytic anemia may develop slowly, with few symptoms. Or it may occur very suddenly, with destruction of half of the total red blood cells in less than thirty minutes. There usually are grave side effects from such a sudden change in the blood's oxygen-carrying capacity, as well as from the problem of trying to dispose of all those damaged red cells now clogging up the circulatory system. This phenomenon is called a hemolytic crisis. Among its causes: the bite of a highly poisonous snake.

A form of hemolytic anemia may occur in newborn children who have a blood type incompatible with the blood type of the mother. In this situation, the red cells of the child may contain an antigen inherited from the father and not present in the blood of the mother. The danger of exposure to new antigens is that they result in the production of defensive antibodies. The mother will, therefore, produce antibodies against this antigen—antibodies which will attack the fetus's red blood cells, and destroy them. Unless treated promptly after birth by means of exchange transfusions, this condition could prove fatal to the child.

---

*Total White Blood Cell Count (WBC)*
Normal range: 5,000 to 10,000 per cubic millimeter

---

In comparison to red blood cells, the number of white blood cells is relatively small. There are approximately 500 times as many reds as there are whites. Yet white blood cells have a crucial and distinct function of their own. They act as our first-line protectors and fighters against infection.

White blood cells have often proved to be headline-makers in today's spectacular transplant technology. Most of us are familiar with the dramatic progress made in overcoming the body's rejection mechanism in heart and other organ transplants. Whether through radiation or drug therapy, what has been done is to suppress or alter some of the white blood cells which normally defend the body against all invaders. A well-known side effect of such anti-rejection therapy has been susceptibility to infection. The challenge now for medical science is to somehow prevent the white blood cells from attacking the alien transplanted organ, without reducing their ability to attack disease-causing intruders.

White blood cells come in a number of different forms, each with a specific function for combating disease. Should your white cell count be either too low or too high, your physician will order a differential count to pinpoint which of your blood cells are responsible for the irregularity. When frequent abnormalities are likely, as in hospitalized patients, a white blood cell differential count may be done as a routine part of the complete blood count.

The total white count is useful to the physician. It is usually elevated during bacterial infections but *not* in viral infections. These elevations may range from 12,000 to 20,000 white blood cells, depending on the severity of the infection and the body's response. Elevations are also found in appendicitis, inflammatory conditions, leukemia, hemolytic anemia of the newborn, and in normal pregnancy. Strenuous exercise, anxiety, and emotional stress can elevate the white cell count.

Among factors which depress the white cell count, viral infections, radiation, and anti-rejection therapy have already been mentioned. Some anti-cancer therapies will have a similar effect, as will rheumatoid arthritis, cirrhosis of the liver, and the less severe form of lupus erythematosus affecting the skin only. In all these conditions, the patient's resistance to bacterial infections is likely to suffer.

The total white count can also be useful to the physician in tracking the progress of infections and certain other diseases in children. During childhood, the response to infections will result in higher white cell elevations than would be expected in adults. Even slight changes in the course of the disease are likely to be reflected in the white blood count. A useful tool, considering that children may not always be able to express their symptoms.

---

*Hemoglobin*
Normal range, at birth: 14 to 23 grams per 100 milliliters (g/100 ml)
Normal range, females: 12 to 16 grams per 100 milliliters
Normal range, males: 14 to 18 grams per 100 milliliters

---

What this test seeks to determine is how much hemoglobin by weight you have in a given quantity of blood.

The result could prove crucial, for hemoglobin is that specific part of your red blood cells which actually does the transporting of oxygen from the lungs to the cells of the body. The production of hemoglobin takes place in the bone marrow as part of the manufacture of red blood cells.

Hemoglobin levels below normal will result in anemia, and the body will simply not have enough oxygen to function effectively.

One of the known causes of a decrease in the production of hemoglobin is the ingestion of lead (which is toxic in other ways as well). Children in old, often substandard housing may eat flakes of old paint high in lead content and end up with lead poisoning as well as anemia. A well-meaning parent may paint a family crib for a new baby and, if not careful, could use leaded paint which the baby could ingest by teething on the railings.

Hemoglobin has also figured prominently in the much-publicized disease called sickle cell anemia. This disease predominantly affects blacks. What happens in sickle cell anemia is that the hemoglobin molecule has been genetically altered, with one amino acid being substituted for the "normal" one. This small alteration (hemoglobin contains three hundred amino acids) causes the red blood cells to assume an irregular shape which is similar to a crescent or a sickle—hence the name—rather than the familiar saucer shape seen in normal individuals. These sickle-shaped cells seem to have a much harder time negotiating their way through the bloodstream than do their normal, well-rounded counterparts. From time to time, the disease erupts in a "sickle cell crisis" as bundles of misshapen cells cause a log jam type of blockage in various blood vessels. This may lead to damage in many organs and disable the patient from pain in the affected areas. Strangely, sickle cell anemia may have begun as an advantageous evolutionary mutation. While people who inherit the sickle cell gene from both parents are likely to die prematurely, those who have only one copy of the gene seem to be unusually resistant to malaria—perhaps the most prevalent as well as the most dangerous disease in the areas where the sickle cell trait is common.

Hemoglobin has also figured prominently, if indirectly, in advertising for iron supplements. What these ads say or imply is that people, especially women, who do not get enough iron may suffer from anemia. This is a valid scientific claim, even if the varied diets of today make this sort of anemia more a thing of the past. The ads are based on the fact that hemoglobin *does* use iron to combine with oxygen; hence, a deficiency of iron in the body will result in a decrease of hemoglobin and, eventually, in anemia when the hemoglobin level falls below the normal range.

When indeed it does occur, iron deficiency anemia can be easily treated with diet or medication containing ferrous iron. The question which should, however, be answered is what caused the decrease in the iron level. Further investigation by the physician is necessary, since not diet but abnormal blood loss may be the ultimate cause.

The normal range for hemoglobin does not leave very much leeway. A condition of anemia is considered to be present when the hemoglobin concentration falls below 14 grams per 100 milliliters for males and 12 grams for females. These sex differences in hemoglobin seem to be due to a specific effect of the principal male hormone, testosterone, in men. However, for all adults over fifty-five, a slight decrease in hemoglobin concentration is normal.

---

*Hematocrit*
Normal range, at birth: 50 to 62 percent
Normal range, males: 40 to 54 percent
Normal range, females: 36 to 46 percent

---

The hematocrit test derives its name from a special capillary tube in which it is performed. The test measures the percentage by volume of red blood cells in whole blood; in other words, the portion of your whole blood that is made up of red blood cells.

Hematocrit is obtained by spinning in a centrifuge a blood sample contained in that special capillary tube. The red blood cells will be packed at the bottom and the clear liquid will be on top. In adult males, the red blood cells should end up filling about half the length of the capillary tube; in adult females, slightly less.

Hematocrit is another measurement of red blood cell mass, taking into account their total volume, which is a product of the number of cells multiplied by their average size. Before modern technology made the red cell count easy and accurate with automatic particle-counting machines, this was the most important and convenient red blood cell test.

A low hematocrit usually indicates anemia. During treatment for anemia, this test is useful for measuring any improvement. As with the red blood cell count, hematocrit can be lower during pregnancy because of increased blood fluids. Hematocrit is also slightly reduced for men over fifty-five years of age.

A high hematocrit is often seen in individuals who are dehydrated or who have an absolute increase in red blood cells, known as polycythemia (see page 82).

---

MCV normal range: 80 to 97 cubic microns ($\mu^3$)
MCH normal range: 27 to 31 picograms (pg)
MCHC normal range: 32 to 36 percent

---

Because of their names, these three tests are often difficult to understand and easy to confuse. Basically, MCV, MCH, and MCHC are used to further define the size of the individual red blood cells and to determine how much oxygen-carrying hemoglobin each cell contains. The results are useful for distinguishing between the various kinds of anemia and in thus determining the correct treatment for individual anemic patients.

MCV reveals the average size of the red blood cells. In technical terms, MCV is the abbreviation for mean corpuscular volume and refers to the relative volume of each red cell. Care must be taken to prevent any delay in analyzing the blood specimen, since the red cells are flexible and can expand by taking in fluid. Enlarged red cells, or those over 97 cubic microns (a micron is one one-thousandth of a millimeter), are referred to as macrocytic; undersized cells, or those below 80 cubic microns, are known as microcytic.

MCH stands for mean corpuscular hemoglobin. MCH actually is not a test but a calculation based on other test results. It seeks to measure the amount of hemoglobin by weight in the average red cell. To calculate it, you divide the hemoglobin result by the number of red blood cells and multiply by 10. For example, if you are a male with a marginal hemoglobin value of 14.0 and your number of red blood cells is 4.7 million, your MCH will be 30 picograms. This puts you close to the upper range of MCH, indicating your red cells have a high oxygen-carrying capacity. If, on the other hand, your red blood cell count rises to 5.4 million while your hemoglobin remains at 14.0, you end up with a subnormal MCH of 26 picograms, suggesting that the oxygen-carrying capacity of individual red blood cells may not be up to par, even though both your hemoglobin and red blood cell count fall within the normal range. MCH thus serves as an extra reassurance—or a warning—when other blood levels seem normal.

MCHC stands for mean corpuscular hemoglobin concentration. What MCHC seeks to measure is the relative volume of hemoglobin in the average red blood cell; in other words, what portion of each red cell is hemoglobin. MCHC, along with MCV, is especially useful in differentiating various anemias.

An abnormally high MCV with MCHC usually greater than 30 percent is associated with pernicious anemia. This anemia is caused by a lack of vitamin $B_{12}$ due to defective absorption of this vitamin from the diet.

An anemia with similar MCV and MCHC findings may develop during pregnancy due to the demand for a greater supply of hemoglobin and red blood cells. In this case, the anemia is caused by a relative deficiency of folic acid, which is a constituent of the B-vitamin complex.

An MCV below 80 and an MCHC below 30 percent are found with iron deficiency anemia, caused by chronic bleeding in the digestive tract or urinary tract, by excessive menstruation, or by repeated pregnancies —which tend to exhaust the iron reserves of the bone marrow—and with some anemias caused by genetic abnormalities.

If the MCV is in the normal range and the MCHC is greater than 30 percent, the following anemias are among the possibilities when hemoglobin or red cell count is also low: hemolytic anemia, blood loss caused by hemophilia, sickle cell anemia, aplastic anemia, and anemias found with various infections, malignancies, and kidney diseases.

## Differential White Cell Count

One purpose of the differential count is to measure the body's capacity to ward off infection. If red and white cell total counts are normal, this test may not be needed. But with an elevation of the total white count, a smear of the blood should be studied to find out which type of white cell is responsible for the overall elevation. With a below-normal white count, a differential count may help to pinpoint specific weaknesses in the body's ability to ward off infection. A second purpose is to evaluate the variations in the different white cells, which may reflect various subtle disease conditions within the body. In the blood stream of normal, healthy individuals, there are six different kinds of white blood cells, each with its own, distinct function:

---

*1. Segmented Neutrophils*
Normal range, adults: 50 to 65 percent
Normal range, children: 25 to 45 percent

---

More than half of the white blood cells in the body are known as segmented neutrophils. They are produced in the bone marrow and take about nine days to mature before they are ready to be released into the bloodstream. For every mature neutrophil released into the blood, there are about twenty immature neutrophils developing in the bone marrow —ready to be released on short notice should infection threaten.

Segmented neutrophils do not spend much time in the bloodstream. Within less than twenty-four hours, they leave it and enter the body's tissues. In the tissues, neutrophils are able to move in large numbers to any site of infection, engulfing the offending bacteria and, in effect, destroying them.

If there is no action for the neutrophils to perform—that is, if there is no infection to combat—the neutrophils will self-destruct about five days after their entry into the tissues. The dead neutrophils will then be eliminated from the body through the saliva, in the intestinal-tract fluids, urine, and bronchial secretions. Some of the dead neutrophils may also be removed by the lymph glands and the spleen.

Increases in segmented neutrophils above normal are most often seen in bacterial infections. The body has mobilized whatever neutrophils are available and thrown them into the front lines. Curiously, bacterial infections may sometimes also *lower* the neutrophil count below normal. This is because neutrophils may leave the bloodstream in large numbers to enter the tissues and move to the site of the infection. And that is where they are, doing their work—rather than in the bloodstream, from which the sample has been drawn. Lower neutrophil counts are most likely to occur at the onset of infections, before the bone marrow has had a chance to step up its production and meet the increased demand from its reserves of maturing neutrophils.

Acute appendicitis and leukemia of the granulocytic type both raise neutrophil levels, but in leukemia the increase in segmented neutrophils is profound. Whereas the total white cell count in most infections rarely jumps to over 20,000, in leukemia the minimum white cell count is usually 50,000—consisting mainly of segmented neutrophils.

Parents sometimes fear that their children who develop shockingly high white cell counts may have leukemia when, in fact, such counts are usually due to an infectious disease. This is because children often have a far more pronounced response to an attack of invading germ cells than do adults. The neutrophil readings may, for a while, approach those for leukemia. But after a few days, the scare usually subsides as the readings fall rapidly and return to normal.

Other causes for an increase in neutrophils may include physiological changes resulting from fear, anger, or exposure to extreme heat or cold; severe exercise; drugs such as digitalis and various corticosteroids; poisons such as arsenic, turpentine, lead, mercury, and benzene; some snake venoms; and carbon monoxide.

A decrease in the level of neutrophils can be caused by many of the same factors that damage all white blood cells or impair their development. Among these are prescription drugs such as colchicine, used for gout; vincristine, procarbazine, or nitrogen mustard, used for tumor therapy; and yes, alcohol when indulged in to excess. In using these life-saving but highly toxic drugs, physicians order frequent white cell counts to forestall any unacceptable damage.

---

### 2. Lymphocytes
Normal range, adults: 25 to 40 percent
Normal range, children: 40 to 60 percent

---

Lymphocytes are the second most common type of white blood cells. Manufactured in the spleen, lymph nodes, and intestinal-related lymph tissue, lymphocytes give immunity primarily against viral diseases by producing neutralizing antibodies.

Lymphocytes protect against such organisms as tuberculosis or brucellosis bacteria. It is lymphocytes that play the main role in rejection of grafts and transplants by identifying them as foreign tissue. This type of lymphocyte has been especially modified by the thymus gland. It is long-lived, remaining in the bloodstream for months and even years.

Because of their longevity, these lymphocytes can sometimes cause severe problems. They are responsible for what is known as delayed hypersensitivity. If, for example, you get stung by a bee, you may not get much of a reaction. But the next time, perhaps years later, the lymphocytes will be ready. They will remember the bee venom as foreign matter and will throw everything into the battle. The result is overreaction, in the form of a sudden release of histamine which may, within minutes, prove fatal to the body the lymphocytes are supposed to be protecting.

Another type of lymphocyte is relatively short-lived, staying in the body only for a matter of days. These are the lymphocytes that form antibodies against various invading viruses. They do their work on demand and then disappear from the scene.

Elevations of such short-lived lymphocytes are usually caused by any number of viral infections, including various forms of the common flu, whooping cough, German measles, and infectious mononucleosis.

A decrease in lymphocytes may result from immune-system deficiencies, increased levels of the pituitary hormone ACTH due to stress, Hodgkin's disease, loss of lymphocytes into the intestinal tract because of blocked drainage from the lymphatic system, and anti-cancer drugs.

Lymphocytes will also decrease dramatically in anti-rejection therapy—leaving the patient highly susceptible to viral and other infectious diseases.

---

*3. Monocytes*
Normal range: 4 to 10 percent

---

Monocytes serve as inflammation fighters. Not very plentiful, they are, however, the largest cells in normal blood. Monocytes are produced in bone marrow, then migrate into the bloodstream, where they remain for about three days before they are ready to migrate into the body's tissues and take up their battle stations.

Monocytes do not do the actual fighting themselves. In the tissues they are transformed into a new cell called a macrophage. In inflammations, macrophages engulf and digest the foreign particles as well as the damaged body cells causing the reaction.

As macrophages, monocytes can live for months in body tissues, prepared to repulse any invasion from outside harmful agents. They can not only do battle against inflammations, but are ready to combat certain bacteria as well as many pollens and viruses. They have the added capability of ingesting stagnant fluids that have collected in the inflamed tissues—and thus help reduce swelling.

A rise in monocytes beyond the normal range can be expected during recovery from many acute infections. Connective-tissue disorders, colitis, and other inflammatory processes may also elevate monocytes. Elevations are sometimes caused by such blood-system disorders as monocytic leukemia, by Hodgkin's disease, and by other disorders of cell growth. A consistent and long-term elevation of monocytes may precede the development of leukemia by months or years.

---

## 4. Eosinophils
Normal range: 1 to 4 percent

---

Although the exact function of eosinophils is not as well defined as that of other white blood cells, their specific task seems to be to protect such tissues as the skin, the lungs, and the gastrointestinal tract. Eosinophils take their name after the red dye eosin, which is used to stain these cells in identifying them.

Eosinophils are made in the bone marrow along with other white blood cells. After their release into the bloodstream, eosinophils migrate into those tissues they are designed to protect—lung, skin, and the gastrointestinal tract—where their concentration is about a hundred times greater than elsewhere. Eosinophils do their work by digesting offending foreign particles by means of an enzyme and other chemicals carried within their cellular structure.

A related aspect of eosinophils at work is their special capability against allergic reactions in the areas which they protect. An allergy represents the body's overreaction through overproduction of antibodies. Eosinophils can digest both the antigen which produces the antibodies as well as the antibodies themselves.

Elevations of eosinophils beyond the normal range can thus be expected during allergic reactions and other illnesses of the organs they protect; for example, in bronchial asthma, in hay fever, in allergic exzema, and in skin reactions to medications. The skin rashes of scarlet fever—which are probably allergic responses to the infection—are also associated with increased eosinophils in the blood. And in the intestinal tract, eosinophils begin to rise soon after infestation with parasites, and remain high for weeks and even months.

Other conditions may also cause a rise in eosinophils. Certain leukemias in which there is a general overstimulation of bone marrow cells will result in elevated eosinophils. This disease is known as eosinophilic leukemia.

Elevated eosinophils may be caused by various drugs and chemicals. For example, the solvent benzene, phosphorus used in industry, and drugs like chlorpromazine may cause allergic-like reactions which result in increased eosinophils.

A decrease in eosinophils is quite common during childbirth, after electric shock therapy, and following the administration of cortisone and related steroids.

---

## 5. Basophils
Normal range: Less than 1 percent

---

Basophils take their name from basic dyes which turn them deep purple and make them easily recognizable on a blood smear.

The least numerous of the white blood cells, basophils are similar in their origin and development to eosinophils and neutrophils.

An increase in basophils is seen during allergic reactions, in polycythemia vera, and in chronic granulocytic leukemia. An elevation is occasionally observed during the chronic breakdown of red blood cells known as hemolytic anemia.

Because of the very low level of basophils in normal individuals, a decrease in basophil count to below normal is difficult to measure—and even more difficult to attribute to a disease condition. As a rule of thumb, a decrease in basophils may parallel situations in which there is a decrease in eosinophils.

---

## 6. Bands
Normal range: 2 percent or less

---

Band cells are actually immature neutrophils. They are normally confined to the bone marrow, where their purpose is to develop into mature neutrophils. But occasionally, during acute infections, bands enter the bloodstream prematurely to help in the fight against the invaders.

An increase in the percentage of band cells, therefore, usually indicates that a high demand has been placed on the body for neutrophils. But an increase in bands can also be the result of an unexplained increase in bone marrow production of white blood cells. Further investigation by the physician is necessary to find a generalized illness that can explain such a change in bone marrow function.

# 7
# More on Your Blood Profile

The following tests are not a part of the routine CBC blood profile your doctor may order as a normal part of an annual physical. These are additional tests which may be needed to explain some abnormalities found in the routine CBC tests. Or the doctor might find them useful for formulating a course of treatment and following up on its effectiveness. These tests give you a chance to take an even closer look at the cells circulating in your blood than do the routine CBC tests.

*Reticulocyte Count*
Normal range: 0.5 to 1.5 percent of total red blood cells

As you may recall, it takes approximately six days for red blood cells to form and enter the bloodstream. Reticulocytes are red cells that have not yet matured and are in the final stages of their six-day development.

The reticulocyte count is important in the diagnosis of various anemias. It tells the doctor at what point the red blood cell deficiency is being caused; whether through a lack of reticulocytes being manufactured in the bone marrow, or through some disorder which prevents them from maturing into full-fledged red blood cells.

In ordering a reticulocyte count, your doctor will most likely also order a fresh hematocrit reading. This will provide a more accurate reticulocyte reading by taking into account any deviation from normal in the hematocrit result. Many laboratories automatically do a hematocrit and make whatever adjustments may be necessary in the result before they send it to the doctor.

How many reticulocytes should you have? Again, you may recall that the expected life span of red cells in your bloodstream varies from 100 to 140 days. That means your bone marrow must replace about 1 percent of the mature red cells in the blood every day. In other words, about 1 percent of your red cells should be in the form of reticulocytes, ready to mature into red blood cells. The normal range gives you ample leeway in either direction.

An elevated reticulocyte count could mean the increased destruction of mature red blood cells, as in hemolytic anemia. The reticulocytes might be there in their normal numbers, but the lower-than-normal mature red cell count would raise the proportion of reticulocytes. Or there might be a true increase in the total number of reticulocytes as a result of the body's attempt to make up for the red blood cell loss. Unsuspected blood loss in the intestinal tract or elsewhere could cause such an increase in reticulocytes. A defect in the production of hemoglobin—as seen in iron deficiency anemia—could also spur the bone marrow to greater reticulocyte production.

Damage to bone marrow by toxic chemicals could cause the bone marrow to malfunction, with either an increase or a decrease in reticulocytes. However, during the course of some cancers, there is likely to be a decrease in the percentage of reticulocytes. Tumor cells may invade and crowd the bone marrow, reducing its capacity to generate reticulocytes as well as mature red blood cells.

If anemia were discovered as part of your CBC screening test, the reticulocyte count could provide your doctor with an added insight into some of the probable causes of this condition.

---

*Platelet Count*
Normal range: 140,000 to 400,000 per cubic millimeter

---

You get a cut or scrape and, most of the time, you do not give it a second thought. In short order, the wound seems to dry up and you are on your way. You may pay even less attention if the injury did not break the skin. You might notice a black-and-blue mark, and that will be the end of the matter. Most persons will even have difficulty recalling how the injury happened.

The reason most of us can be so carefree about occasional cuts, scrapes, and bruises is because our clotting mechanism is working smoothly. The clotting mechanism is one of the body's most complex functions. More than a dozen different factors are involved, none of which is more important than the role played by the smallest cell particles in the blood, known as platelets.

When the body is wounded or cut, the platelets react by forming clumps and sticking together at breaks in the tiniest blood vessels. They form a temporary plug which stops the outflow of blood and is eventually replaced by a more permanent clot. The clot is also formed partly from platelets—plus fibrin strands developed by the action of multiple clotting factors in the blood.

In the case of a bruise, platelets act like a sort of instant glue. What happens when skin tissue is bruised is that a blow has damaged capillary walls and blood is seeping out into the surrounding tissues. The platelets become adhesive and soon seal up the break in the capillary walls to stop further loss of blood into the tissues.

About one-third of the body's supply of platelets are stored in the spleen. If the spleen is removed, these platelets will remain in the bloodstream. People without spleens may have as many as a million platelets per cubic millimeter of blood.

Such an elevation is not usually considered dangerous. However, other elevations over the upper limit of normal could be a reaction to blood loss due to hemorrhage, or a breakdown of red blood cells, as in hemolytic anemia. Elevated levels of platelets are also seen in inflammatory diseases, in certain malignancies, and in polycythemia vera.

Decreased platelet levels are an important aid in the diagnosis of bleeding disorders. The causes for a decreased platelet count can be several; but all are of serious concern to the physician. People with decreased platelets are exposed to the danger of bleeding in the brain, which can result in neurologic damage or even death.

Decreased platelet levels can be caused by poor platelet production. This is often the case with anemias related to vitamin $B_{12}$, or folic acid, deficiencies, and in cases of damage to bone marrow tissue, as in aplastic anemia.

Another cause for decreased platelet count is that the body has mistakenly destroyed the platelets through its antibody defense mechanism. This unfortunate situation can be triggered by such drugs as quinidine, sulfa drugs, or barbiturates. The platelets become involved in the body's response against these drugs and are inadvertently destroyed in the combat between the drugs and their antibodies. Newborn babies are sometimes affected by similar platelet destruction, caused by the antibodies of the mother prior to birth.

Reduced levels of platelets often are a cause of a condition known as petechiae, or tiny red spots which appear all over the body and usually become purple. They are a form of bleeding into the skin, and can be symptomatic of a major blood disease, perhaps even leukemia. However, a very hot and brisk shower can sometimes bring out a similar sprinkling of spots. These may be frightening but are really nothing to worry about.

People taking two aspirin or other salicylate-containing preparations may be in for a similar scare. Their platelet count and ability to form clots may be normal, but their protection from hemorrhage remains inadequate. This is because salicylates prevent large clumps of platelets from coming together the way they normally do. As these people continue taking aspirin or similar salicylate medications, their bodies may become increasingly marked by those scary little red spots. Shortly after the salicylate-containing medication is discontinued, the condition fades away.

This special capability of aspirin to keep platelets from clumping together has recently been put to good use for high-cholesterol, high-triglyceride patients who are in danger of forming blood clots. Blood clots occur when deposits of cholesterol in the arteries become coated with triglycerides and are further enlarged by the addition of large clumps of platelets. Four aspirins a day seem to lower the chances of these clumps of platelets ever coming together in sufficient numbers to form a blood clot. Salicylate-containing drugs are thus becoming an important adjunct in the campaign against strokes and heart attacks.

---

*Prothrombin Time*

Therapy range: To be determined by attending physician. Patients on anticoagulant or clot prevention therapy are usually maintained in the 60 to 70 percent range and rarely allowed to fall below 50 percent of normal. For those not on therapy, anything less than 100 percent could be abnormal. Results are usually reported as a time ratio for the patient's clot formation against the normal control.

---

To anyone susceptible to blood clots, knowing about prothrombin time could be a matter of life and death. Prothrombin time is a measure of the time it takes for a clot to form in a patient's blood compared to normal blood. The main reason for this test is to monitor the therapy of individuals receiving anti-clotting drugs. The idea is to give enough of such medication to the patients—who have had heart attacks or strokes or have blood clots in their veins—to keep further clots from forming. At the same time, the doctor must be careful not to inhibit blood clot formation to such an extent that uncontrolled bleeding could develop.

The drugs used are the various coumarin compounds, including the most popular one, coumadin. To give you an idea of how critically the dosage must be watched, coumarin is the same ingredient that goes into many rat poisons. These rat poisons work by interfering with blood clotting to such an extent that the rats soon die of internal bleeding.

The clotting mechanism is very complicated. At least twelve different factors are involved, including platelets, described in the previous section. Some of the other clotting factors are made in the liver, with the help of vitamin K. What coumarin drugs do is to compete with vitamin K's activity in the liver, thus reducing some of the essential clotting factors that are produced there.

Prothrombin time also has a vital use for patients who are not on any blood-thinning therapy but who are prone to hemorrhages. Normal blood will clot in approximately twelve or thirteen seconds. Any significant increase above thirteen seconds is usually a cause for concern; clotting is taking too long and hemorrhaging may result.

If the prothrombin time is abnormal, the doctor will suspect that four clotting factors may be responsible; namely, those that have been labeled II, V, VII, and X. There are several other tests which can specifically pinpoint the other individual factors among another eight clotting factors that may be causing the problem.

What causes these deficiencies in clotting? Medical science does not yet have all the answers. To begin with, various liver diseases or a deficiency in vitamin K can affect the production of one or more of the clotting factors. And this could happen at any age. Some of the causes may be genetic. In those cases, the body's inability to make enough of the specific clotting factor will probably make itself known shortly after birth. Robert K. Massie's best-selling book and popular film *Nicholas and Alexandra* dramatized the heartbreak when such a condition afflicted the son of the Czar of Russia. As a hemophiliac, the young Czarevich was missing factor VII. How simple and straightforward it all seems today. Yet the Czarina's involvement with the infamous Rasputin in her search for a cure was one of the factors which caused the downfall of the Romanov dynasty—and changed history forever!

Today, hemophilia and other clotting disorders need not necessarily be the cause of unmitigated tragedy. With prothrombin time and various other tests, the physician can identify the components causing the bleeding, and has increasingly better methods to correct the problem.

## Erythrocyte Sedimentation Rate (ESR)

*Erythrocyte Sedimentation Rate (ESR)*
Normal range, males: Less than 15 millimeters per hour
Normal range, females: Less than 20 millimeters per hour
Normal range, males over 50: Less than 20 millimeters per hour
Normal range, females over 50: Less than 30 millimeters per hour

This is another one of those very basic tests which answers the questions: Are you ill? And if so, are you better today than yesterday, or are you worse?

What ESR measures is the speed at which red blood cells will settle from whole, unclotted blood in a special tube designed for that purpose. The relationship between the rate of settling and many disease conditions has been known for a long time. In general, the slower the cells settle— that is, the shorter the distance they travel downward within an hour— the less chance there is of disease; or the greater the degree of improvement for the patient.

The reason ESR will increase during some diseases is that the body makes increased levels of fibrinogen and globulin proteins. This will tend to make the red blood cells sticky, binding them together like a roll of wrapped coins. Since they are now heavier than normal individual cells, these rolls of cells—appropriately called rouleaux bodies—will settle faster in plasma than do normal cells.

The size of the red cell itself can affect the rate of settling. In certain anemias, the cells may become larger than normal. Consequently, they will settle faster, being heavier than normal cells. The ESR may also increase if the total number of cells is decreased. This is because the remaining cells will meet less resistance and jostling from other cells on their way to the bottom.

Just about the only benign conditions which can lead to increased ESR are menstruation and pregnancy. Starting in about their third month, pregnant women will usually have an increased sedimentation rate, which will fall back to normal about a month after delivery.

Among the abnormal conditions which are known to increase the settling rate of red blood cells are tuberculosis, cancer, heart attacks, rheumatoid and other types of arthritis, rheumatic fever, acute hepatitis, thyroid disorders, kidney damage, acute inflammation, and blood protein disorders such as multiple myeloma. None of the above can be taken lightly; so, unless you are menstruating or pregnant at the time of this test, an increased sedimentation rate calls for further investigation of the cause. One caution: this test must be done with a freshly drawn specimen to provide a meaningful answer.

## About Your Blood Type

Blood typing has become a very sophisticated and sometimes very delicate science. Called upon to determine the paternity of a set of fraternal twins, one of the world's top experts in the field came to the hard-to-believe conclusion that each of the twins had a different father. How to broach the subject with the mother—not to speak of the two fathers—without being called a medical fraud? Much to this expert's relief, the mother readily confirmed that yes, dual fatherhood was indeed a possibility!

Most people will probably never have occasion to require that kind of detailed blood typing—and would probably just as soon skip it. The kind of blood typing we are talking about is relatively simple. If you have ever donated or received blood, had an operation in a hospital, or served in the armed forces, the chances are you have already had your blood typed in this manner.

The purpose of blood typing is to prevent blood-group incompatibilities. Blood typing ensures that patients do not get the wrong type of blood, which could cause serious side effects and even death. Blood typing can also prevent complications in newborns whose blood type is incompatible with that of the mother.

Blood typing is necessary because all red blood cells and other cells of your body contain unique characteristics on their surfaces, caused by slight differences in their chemical composition. These differences are sufficiently unique so that the body can detect those that are not its very own.

Your blood-group components are genetically determined and inherited from your parents. More than fifty such characteristics have been identified so far, but the principal groups are called A, B, AB, and O. In the United States, approximately 45 percent of the population has blood type O; 41 percent, type A; 10 percent, type B; and 4 percent, type AB.

Many people believe in being ready for any emergency. They carry their blood type engraved on a bracelet or as a part of their identification papers. There is good reason for it.

Let us say you are blood type A. What would happen if you were mistakenly given a transfusion of type B blood? A mild reaction might set in almost instantly. This is because there is a good chance that your blood would, as a matter of course, already contain some antibodies against type B blood. Moreover, your body would quickly recognize the type B blood as foreign and would start manufacturing additional antibodies against it. These antibodies would make every attempt to destroy the foreign red blood cells—giving you a fever and diverse pains.

It would be even worse if you were given *another* transfusion of type B blood, perhaps months or years later. This time, your body would be even better prepared to attack the invader. It would react on a more massive scale, completely destroying the red cells given in this second transfusion. Not only would the fever and pain be more intense, but the destruction of such large numbers of red cells would release unmanageable amounts of hemoglobin, which could prove highly toxic to your body and possibly destroy your kidney function.

But typing your blood for A, B, and O groups is not enough to assure safe transfusions. There is another special substance found on the surface of red blood cells of some people. It is called the Rh factor. Approximately 80 percent of our population have it in their blood. They are known as Rh-positive; the others are Rh-negative.

Rh-positive cells transfused into Rh-negative blood are capable of triggering the production of massive quantities of antibodies that will attack and destroy the Rh-positive cells. Rh-negative cells do not trigger a similar reaction in Rh-positive blood, because they do not contain any Rh factor to act as an antigen.

It is therefore relatively safe to give Rh-negative blood to an Rh-positive person. But the reverse could prove highly dangerous. If you happened to be Rh-negative, giving you Rh-positive blood would leave you open to a response similar to what could happen to the person with type A blood who is given that *second* transfusion of type B blood. Your body would react violently, breaking up all the invading Rh-positive cells —and leaving you in a very serious condition.

In pregnancy, the Rh factor can be of special concern. If the mother is Rh-negative and her first child is Rh-positive, the chances are that some of the child's Rh-positive cells entered the mother's bloodstream during delivery. This usually happens when the afterbirth material, or placenta, is disconnected from the uterus. The newborn is fine and so is the mother. But the mother begins making antibodies against the Rh-positive cells from the baby. She becomes sensitized to that blood-group factor. In a subsequent pregnancy, if the unborn child is again Rh-positive, then the antibodies of the sensitized mother can cross the placental lining and attack the baby's red blood cells. The baby may be stillborn or anemic.

Doctors can now prevent this danger in subsequent pregnancies by taking steps in the first pregnancy. Shortly after delivery, they inject the mother with a substance called RhoGam. RhoGam contains antibodies against the child's Rh-positive blood that has been introduced into the mother's system. These antibodies eliminate the Rh-positive cells so fast that the mother's own defense system never has the need to go to work. She thus avoids becoming sensitized against the Rh-positive factor of some future child that she may carry.

Even when the Rh factor has been properly identified and the red cells correctly typed, blood transfusions can sometimes still cause reactions. There are, in fact, more than fifty different reactive factors that have already been discovered in the blood of various people. Some are named after the families where they were first identified: Duffy, Kell, Kidd, Lewis. Others carry less memorable designations, such as M and N. Rarely will any of these minor factors cause reactions of the severity expected from Rh or blood-group incompatibilities. But the possibility of an unusual reaction is always there.

Blood banks take elaborate precautions to prevent such reactions through a process called cross-matching. In addition to establishing the Rh factor and the major A, B, and O typing, a selected number of minor factors are also checked in the blood of both donor and recipient. Also checked is the presence of any antibodies against the various red cell characteristics in either of the two specimens. Although it is difficult to get a perfect match of all the minor characteristics—and a total absence of antibodies—the idea is to come as close as possible.

Closely related to blood cross-matching is tissue typing. The fast-growing field of organ transplantation would be impossible without tissue typing. This developing new science seeks to identify tissue cell characteristics that are inherited in much the same way as the various factors on the surface of red blood cells. If there are too many differences between the cells of donor and recipient tissues, the transplant will be rejected. The closer the match, the easier it will be to control the body's rejection mechanism.

It is perhaps in paternity suits that tissue and blood typing come together to meet one of their most interesting challenges. Given the tissue and blood characteristics of the mother and child, the various candidates for fatherhood can often be narrowed down to one. It is usually far easier to prove that an individual is not the father than that he is, since all it takes to disprove paternity is to find one factor that does not fit.

# 8
# Hormones: The Body's Messengers

Have you ever considered the complexities of keeping the different parts of your body working in unison? Never mind the billions of cells which have to be individually fed, cleansed, and otherwise nurtured. But consider for a moment the enormity of the task of just keeping the major organs in touch with each other and coordinating their activities. The brain, the intestinal tract, the heart and blood vessels, the liver and pancreas, the kidneys, testes, ovaries: complex as they are in themselves, they have to work together in a fine-tuned and synchronous manner if you are to be able to fulfill your daily tasks.

What helps keep your body in such an integrated state is a communications network that is second to none. This network enables specialized glands to control other glands, to adjust the function of body tissues, and to monitor the chemical state of the entire body. This internal system is able to maintain the delicate balance typical of a healthy person in the same way that a thermostat adjusts the temperature in a house.

Your body's communications network actually is made up of two separate systems. The one with which most people are most familiar is the nervous system. This is a network of nerve cells and specialized nerve fibers, receiving and sending throughout the body countless messages which are processed by the most remarkable of all control centers, the brain.

The endocrine system is more subtle and less familiar. It works on the basis of minuscule amounts of hormones, highly specialized chemicals which are released in one part of the body and selectively delivered to action sites in remote areas.

Along with vitamins, hormones today are probably among the most talked-about components of the body. Not only are they known for their amazing healing properties in such traditional areas as skin disorders and eye diseases, but people often ascribe to them near-magical powers in newer fields. Some women want them for birth control and others for increased fertility. Men may look to hormones to restore their sexual performance or increase their athletic potential.

It could perhaps be said that as part of our drug culture, we have also developed a hormone culture. As people learn more about the powers of hormones, they may become eager to use hormones beyond the limits found safe by medical scientists. With more knowledge of how hormones do their work, people might be more cautious and respectful in their usage.

The hormones found naturally in the body are manufactured by groups of specialized glands in widely separated locations. These glands include the pituitary, at the base of the brain; the thyroid and parathyroid glands, in the front, lower part of the neck; the adrenal glands, which are near the top surface of each of the kidneys; the pancreas, located just behind the stomach; the ovaries, next to the uterus; and the testicles, within the scrotum. Collectively, they are known as the endocrine glands, and the study of their structure and functions is called endocrinology.

In fulfilling their communications role between organs, hormones function like chemical switches. By increasing chemical activity, they can turn on or increase certain biological functions and turn off or decrease other functions which are not required at that moment. The word "hormone" is derived from the Greek, meaning to excite or stimulate.

The master control gland in the body is the pituitary. Only somewhat larger than a pea, this gland is controlled directly by the brain. The pituitary's activity is extremely complex. The gland is known to secrete at least eight different chemical substances, each with its own specific set of functions on widely separated organs throughout the body.

In contrast, the parathyroid glands secrete only one hormone, with one basic function—to maintain the proper balance of calcium in the body. Most of the other glands, on the scale of versatility, fall somewhere between the pituitary and the parathyroid glands.

Since endocrine glands have no ducts, their secretions are passed directly into the bloodstream as it flows through them. The bloodstream then circulates these hormones in their minute quantities throughout the body, enabling the target organs to identify the hormone, measure the amount, and respond appropriately.

Virtually all hormones are formed in such small amounts that until recent years laboratories could not accurately make these delicate measurements that the body does continuously as a matter of course. After all, how do you weigh something that is measured in billionths or trillionths of a gram?

The answer has come with a technique known as radioimmunoassay. Developed in the 1960s, this technique makes possible the accurate measurement of hormones in a blood sample through radioactive labeling, and then measuring the amount of radiation. It is a fairly complex process but one which can give you the results in one to three days at a cost ranging from ten to one hundred dollars, depending on the hormone tested.

With radioimmunoassay, hormone levels can be measured either in the blood or the urine. But except for total estrogens, blood samples are far more frequently used than urine samples. This is because the urine measurement is based on the amounts of hormone produced in a twenty-four-hour sample of urine. Most people find it inconvenient to collect the urine and then carry it over to the doctor's office for shipment to a laboratory. With the predicted development of even more sensitive blood tests for hormones, urine tests for hormones are fast becoming a thing of the past.

---

*Blood Constituents: Thyroid Hormones $T_4$ and $T_3$*

Normal range, total $T_4$: 5.0 to 13.0 micrograms per 100 milliliters (mcg/100ml)

Normal range, free $T_4$: 0.8 to 2.4 nanograms per 100 milliliters (ng/100ml)

Normal range, total $T_3$: 50 to 200 nanograms per 100 milliliters (ng/100 ml)

Normal range, $T_3$ uptake: 30 to 40 percent

---

In the words of Madison Avenue: Do you often feel tired, sluggish, listless? Or restless, excitable, irritable? If so, your thyroid gland might not be functioning property. The tests for thyroid-gland activity are among those most commonly performed today. Some physicians even include thyroid function as a part of the routine screening tests.

Located in the front part of the neck, the thyroid gland occupies a key position as the prime regulator of the body's metabolic activity. It serves somewhat like the gas pedal of your car, determining how fast or how slow your system will function—from digesting the food you eat to processing the thoughts you have.

Two thyroid gland hormones known as $T_4$ and $T_3$ are responsible for ensuring that your body functions at the proper speed. How this is done is a very delicate and complex process.

To begin with, in order for your thyroid gland to manufacture these two active hormones, you must have an adequate supply of iodine in your diet. Traditionally, seafood has been the main source of dietary iodine. Until recently, there were many people in the United States, and especially in land-locked countries abroad, who were not getting enough iodine. In trying to compensate for this deficiency, their thyroid glands would enlarge and develop the condition known as goiter. Today, with the regular addition of iodine to table salt, most people get enough of this vital mineral in their normal diet.

The thyroid gland acts like a magnet to attract traces of iodine from within the body. In the thyroid gland, the iodine combines, to different degrees, with an amino acid called tyrosine. Some of the tyrosine units end up with one iodine molecule, some with two molecules, some with three, and others with four. When the tyrosine units have acquired as many as three or four iodine molecules, they become the active thyroid hormones known in the trade as $T_4$ and $T_3$, reflecting the number of iodine molecules each possesses. $T_4$ is far more plentiful than $T_3$, but $T_3$ is far more powerful than $T_4$. $T_4$ is also commonly referred to as thyroxine.

As they are produced, the $T_3$ and $T_4$ hormones are stored in the thyroid gland. When the need for them arises, the brain sends a message to the pituitary gland, which in turn relays the message to the thyroid gland by releasing the thyroid-stimulating hormone, TSH.

TSH causes the thyroid gland to release its stores of ready-made $T_4$ and $T_3$ hormones into the bloodstream. At the same time, the thyroid gland begins to manufacture additional $T_4$ and $T_3$ hormones to replace those that have been called into action.

In the bloodstream, most $T_3$ and $T_4$ hormones become bound to the carrier proteins. While traveling to different parts of the body, the bound hormones are not able to do any work. Only a small proportion of the $T_3$ and $T_4$ hormones will reach their final destination, freed from the carrier proteins that brought them there and ready for work. These active hormones are known as free $T_3$ and free $T_4$. The combined amounts of bound and free hormones make up the total $T_3$ and total $T_4$ values.

Is it necessary to measure total as well as free $T_4$ and total $T_3$ plus what is known as $T_3$ uptake to test your thyroid-gland function?

All these measurements are not, in fact, always necessary. The best single measurement is free $T_4$. It is a better indicator than total $T_4$ because free $T_4$ measures only the $T_4$ hormone that is available in active form. But until recently, most laboratories were not able to measure free $T_4$ accurately because of the very minute quantities involved, measured in billionths of a gram.

How about total $T_3$? This measurement is sometimes necessary in mysterious cases of overactive thyroid function in which the total $T_4$ and even free $T_4$ tests are not high enough to make a diagnosis despite signs of weight loss, rapid pulse, and tremor of the hands. Such patients represent less than 5 percent of all cases of thyroid-gland overactivity and have a condition called "$T_3$ toxicosis." This problem leads the physician on a merry chase until the total $T_3$ measurement is made and reveals the malfunction. There is also a complicated method to measure free $T_3$, but it is costly and rarely needed.

As for $T_3$ uptake, it is not a test for $T_3$ in the blood but an indirect measure of the amount of carrier protein available to thyroid hormones in the bloodstream. Before the new free $T_4$ test, $T_3$ uptake was used along with total $T_4$ to estimate free $T_4$. Obviously, this measurement is no longer necessary now that there is a way to measure free $T_4$ directly. Again, it is the free $T_4$ which is the important measurement.

What if your $T_4$ levels are outside the normal range? People with levels that are above normal are referred to as hyperthyroid; those with values below normal, as hypothyroid. Each has different symptoms and different causes.

In our society, hypothyroidism is much more common than hyperthyroidism, especially in young women. People with hypothyroidism tend to be sluggish, with little or no pep and energy. They are likely to become overweight and have a lackadaisical attitude toward life. These symptoms are caused by lowered metabolic activity, which eventually involves the brain and may lead to a state of confusion and mental incapacity called dementia.

Hypothyroidism is often accompanied by various blood chemistry abnormalities. Fasting blood sugar levels may be subnormal and cholesterol levels abnormally high. Anemia, with oversize individual blood cells, may develop, resembling the changes seen in vitamin $B_{12}$ deficiency, pernicious anemia. Even jaundice may occur, most likely due to the sluggish performance of the liver cells deprived of the spark plug effects of thyroid hormone.

Adults can develop hypothyroidism if their thyroid gland has been surgically removed as treatment for goiter, thyroid cancer, or various tumors. Delayed damage can result from head or neck radiation during childhood. Or the thyroid gland can be damaged when the body for unknown reasons suddenly develops antibodies against the thyroid. Called Hashimoto's thyroiditis, this disorder is indeed common among Oriental people but is also the most prevalent thyroid disease in all countries.

Sometimes hypothyroidism is temporary, due to a lack of iodine in the diet, use of certain medications for treatment of asthma, and various other prescription drugs. Usually, once the cause is removed, the resilient thyroid gland is able to recover its normal function.

Newborns can also suffer from hypothyroidism. As a serious congenital defect, this condition can have tragic results if undiagnosed. The infant will become mentally retarded with a syndrome known as cretinism. There is no way to tell whether a newborn is afflicted with hypothyroidism except by testing. Many hospitals are now doing $T_4$ tests as a matter of routine on all newborns, and if the result is low, an elevated TSH assay will confirm the diagnosis. Treatment must be started within the first ninety days of life in order to prevent lifetime mental retardation.

Hypothyroidism sometimes is not caused by the thyroid gland but by improper circuitry elsewhere. This happens when the pituitary gland fails to receive a proper signal to send out the thyroid stimulating hormone, TSH. In the absence of TSH, the thyroid gland simply will not get the message that the body needs more thyroid hormones. The situation is analogous to one where a home remains unheated because the thermostat is turned off.

If this condition is suspected, the doctor will order a check on TSH levels. Above-normal TSH indicates that the problem is with the thyroid gland, since the pituitary will be prompted to send out additional TSH in an effort to goad the sluggish thyroid gland into action. However, when the problem is with the brain–pituitary–thyroid circuitry, TSH levels will fail to rise out of the normal range.

As one might expect, TSH levels will fall below normal in the opposite condition, hyperthyroidism. The body supply of too much $T_3$ and $T_4$ hormones forces the hypothalamus to slow its production of TRH, thyrotropin-releasing hormone, and the pituitary stops sending

TSH to the thyroid gland. Despite the dwindling supply of TSH, the thyroid gland will continue to produce excessive quantities of $T_3$ and $T_4$. It will be like a thermostat that has been set too high. In fact, the excess of thyroid hormones does generate more body heat and more perspiration.

The symptoms of hyperthyroidism at first make the patient feel very energetic, only to fall into a state of exhaustion later. There is often a tremor of the hands, warm skin with perspiration, and, possibly, heart palpitations. As the body's metabolic rate accelerates, many blood constituents are affected.

Blood sugar levels may increase until sugar appears in the urine. A substance called creatine, essential to good muscle tone, spills into the urine. There may be increased bone breakdown, resulting in elevated levels of calcium in both blood and urine. Liver function may be impaired to such an extent that cholesterol production will fall below normal, insufficient to meet the body's needs for the synthesis of steroid hormones.

What causes the thyroid gland to run out of control? Only rarely is this condition due to thyroid nodules or cancer; usually, there is a general enlargement of the thyroid gland. Hyperthyroidism without a tumor is called Graves' disease. Graves' disease is treated either by medication, by a dose of radioactive iodine, or by the surgical removal of most of the thyroid gland. While the exact cause is uncertain, it is believed that antibodies form and attach to the thyroid gland cells causing a false signal which stimulates the synthesis of thyroid hormones.

Hypothyroidism and hyperthyroidism are serious conditions that are alarmingly prevalent in our society. The various $T_4$ and $T_3$ tests are essential for proper diagnosis to ensure appropriate treatment at the earliest opportunity. Yet the disease itself sometimes interferes with making an early diagnosis. One famous example is that of a physician who had discovered cases of low thyroid function in women who had hemorrhages during childbirth and suffered oxygen lack and damage to the pituitary gland. Dr. H. L. Sheehan, whose name is applied to this rare condition, sent out inquiries requiring the return of a postcard. Those with this slow-thyroid condition failed to reply. They were too sluggish to even reply when asked about their health.

*Blood constituent: Aldosterone*
Normal range, supine: 10 to 100 picograms per milliliter (pg/ml)
Normal range, upright: 30 to 300 picograms per milliliter

The purpose of this test is to evaluate the salt hormone system of your adrenal glands. For people with high blood pressure, this test can also provide clues to certain causes of their condition.

Aldosterone is a steroid compound manufactured in the adrenal glands, located just above each kidney. The main function of this hormone is to regulate the concentration of salt in our bodies and maintain a proper balance of sodium and potassium in order to sustain normal blood volume and to adjust blood pressure.

When the amount of sodium in the blood is too low, blood pressure is not sustained. The ebb of this internal tide results in a call for aldosterone which is speedily released from the adrenal glands. The aldosterone increases the retention of sodium by the kidneys in exchange for potassium which is discarded in the urine. Since water follows wherever sodium goes, there is a net retention of water that restores blood volume and pressure to normal.

An excess level of potassium can directly act on the adrenal glands to trigger an increased secretion of aldosterone which brings about a net loss of potassium in the urine. When the supply of sodium is low, the restoration process is far more complex. A substance called renin is first released by the kidneys. The renin is able to break loose a fragment of ten amino acids from a larger molecule in the blood. The substance is called angiotensin I, which, in turn, is cut down to a chain of eight amino acids called angiotensin II. It is the angiotensin II which acts on the adrenal gland to release the aldosterone.

This complex process explains the mechanism of blood pressure control. Angiotensin II, as the name suggests, acts as a powerful constrictor of your arteries. If renin is overproduced by your kidneys, an excessive amount of angiotensin II will be formed. Result? Constriction of the arteries and elevated blood pressure.

At the same time, the resulting increase in aldosterone will make the body reabsorb more salt—and along with it, more water. By increasing the volume of liquids in the cells and bloodstream, the blood pressure rise will be sustained. This is why people whose high blood pressure is related to an overproduction of renin must be especially careful to restrict their intake of salt. Fortunately, the medication propanolol can block renin production to some extent, and provide relief.

But overproduction of renin is not the sole cause of excessive aldosterone production. Tumors and other disorders in the adrenal gland itself may be responsible for the condition. That is why the physician will include a renin test in order to learn whether the kidneys are at fault or whether the source of the problem lies entirely within the adrenal glands.

Whatever the cause of excess aldosterone, it usually causes extraction of potassium from body cells and fluids. This often shows up on blood tests for electrolytes, which are routine for high blood pressure patients. Low potassium levels can be serious indeed, with muscular cramps, heart weakness, and even death as the result. Low potassium, high sodium, and high blood pressure found in association with high aldosterone levels tend to implicate the adrenal glands in this type of disorder.

Special care must be taken in the interpretation of aldosterone tests, since they can be influenced by diuretics, female hormones, and even by the high blood pressure itself. There is also a special situation in which a patient who is suspected of high aldosterone because of the typical symptoms of low potassium, high sodium, and high blood pressure will have no such thing. This person will have merely indulged in an excess of licorice, which contains a natural substance that acts on the kidneys in a way very similar to aldosterone, and can substitute so completely for it that the body's production is halted. A careful cross-examination by the doctor for "licorice abuse" solves the mystery. The usual amounts taken as a treat are not enough to cause this problem.

An even greater challenge to diagnostic ability is presented by the patients with bizarre behavior involving concealed vomiting or overuse of laxatives. In some cases, the psychiatrists have found that the person is seeking attention from relatives or friends by reducing weight to achieve a fashion-model type of beauty. Sometimes, a plummeting potassium level may attract attention. One such woman became paralyzed by the lack of potassium and was taken by ambulance to an emergency unit, where intravenous potassium solution revived her. The clue to her problem was that no potassium appeared in the urine. It had all been lost by secretive vomiting.

As is often the case, this woman was relieved to be discovered, since she was not able to stop the vomiting and feared to confess that it all started as a ruse. With psychiatric help, she was able to realize that her goals had become misdirected, and eventually recovered completely.

Laboratory tests, including findings of low aldosterone levels, saved her from surgery, since an adrenal tumor was at first suspected. This is another example of the detective function of diagnostic tests.

---

*Blood constituent: Cortisol*
Normal range, morning: 5 to 25 micrograms per 100 milliliters
   (mcg/100ml)

---

The purpose of this test is to check if there are any problems with a major function of the adrenal or pituitary glands. The blood specimen should be drawn early in the morning, but fasting is not necessary. Normal values for specimens drawn in the evening are considerably lower.

Cortisol is another one of the body's vital constituents that is manufactured from cholesterol. Also known as hydrocortisone, it is made by the outer portion of the adrenal glands. Cortisol is very active biologically and makes up about 50 percent of the assorted steroid hormones that are manufactured by the adrenals. The control hormone is called ACTH (adrenocorticotrophic hormone). It is released by the pituitary as a messenger to the adrenal glands to start cortisol production.

Cortisol has a number of different functions which help your body to run smoothly. It acts as a control on blood sugar levels by preventing insulin from removing too much sugar from the bloodstream. When such a situation threatens, cortisol can counteract the action of insulin. At the same time, cortisol can get more glucose into the bloodstream by releasing glucose from its storage depots in the liver and stimulating the liver to manufacture more from protein sources.

Cortisol plays an important role in how the body makes various proteins and fats. Normal cortisol levels are responsible for helping mold the body into its natural shape, with enough muscles and not too much fat. An excess of cortisol could cause undue protein breakdown in the muscles and an excessive buildup of fat around the midriff and other parts of the torso.

You may be familiar with cortisol through its close derivative, cortisone, which was the first miracle drug used to reduce the severe swelling and inflammation of rheumatoid arthritis. The biological effect of cortisol or cortisone is to reduce the migration of white blood cells into the area where the body has been damaged or invaded. You will recall that your white blood cells are the first line of defense against infection.

What often happens is that the body overreacts, sending in more white blood cells than may be necessary, and that causes the inflammation. By keeping the number of white blood cells down, cortisol reduces the intensity of the battle to more manageable proportions. Cortisol and its synthetic substitutes have been used to treat inflammatory conditions of the eyes and skin, as well as hypersensitive reactions to certain drugs or even poison ivy.

Because the reduction in white blood cells lowers the body's ability to fight infections, cortisone must be used with caution in the presence of infections. An antibiotic is usually included to make up for the loss in the body's natural defenses if infection is detected.

If the adrenal glands do not produce enough cortisol because they are damaged or fail to respond to ACTH from the pituitary gland, a serious condition called Addison's disease may develop. The symptoms include loss of appetite, loss of weight, frequent diarrhea, general weakness, low resistance to infection, and anemia. There might even be abnormal pigmentation, whereby the skin takes on a deep bronze coloration. The skin creases, and gums and nipples will darken unless cortisone treatment is given.

Addison's disease can be controlled by cortisone or similar medication. It has often been said that President Kennedy had Addison's disease. The swollen appearance occasionally noted in his face was reportedly due to more than the usual amount of cortisone medication, since he also had an inflammatory condition of the spine which responded to extra cortisone. Such side effects can be avoided by taking only the necessary amount for normal activity.

Cushing's disease is the opposite condition: too much cortisol in the body. The excessive amount of cortisol may be caused by too much ACTH released from a small tumor of the pituitary gland. The surplus ACTH overstimulates the adrenal secretion of cortisol. Or a tumor may form in one of the adrenal glands, resulting in uncontrolled cortisol output by the tumor.

A person with Cushing's disease—or a person treated with high doses of cortisone-type medication—will have problems such as hypertension, loss of sex functions, diabetes, acne, and excessive growth of body hair. Fat will accumulate on the face, buttocks, and lower abdomen, often causing stretch marks. Sometimes there is a purple, mottled discoloration of the lower legs and a facial flush.

It is easy to measure cortisol in conveniently small blood samples. Results are usually ready in one day. If more information is needed, your doctor may order a test of your response to a single injection of synthetic ACTH. Samples taken thirty and sixty minutes after the dose will show how well your adrenal glands respond to a sudden demand for cortisol. A lack of response is typical of adrenal disease or atrophy. An exuberant response is suggestive of Cushing's disease. If the latter condition is suspected, a more detailed study is done by giving one or more doses of dexamethasone, a synthetic substitute for cortisol. This preparation will stop normal adrenal production of cortisol but will fail to stop the excessive secretion prevalent in Cushing's disease. The more complicated tests are generally done under the supervision of an endocrinologist.

---

*Blood constituent: Parathyroid Hormone (PTH)*
Normal range: Dependent on reference laboratory's procedures

---

The purpose of this test is to find out the reasons for any calcium abnormalities in your bloodstream. Regulating the amount of calcium in your blood is the parathyroid hormone's primary function.

Located in the neck region near the thyroid gland, the four parathyroid glands are very sensitive to low levels of calcium. Another hormone called calcitonin, made in specialized "C" cells of the adjacent thyroid gland, is sensitive to high levels of calcium in the bloodstream. The two systems act to control upper and lower limits of blood calcium.

When the parathyroid glands detect subnormal levels of calcium, they begin to release PTH, which acts to bring the calcium level back to normal in three ways:

First, PTH draws upon the reservoir of solid calcium contained in the skeletal bones and causes it to return to the bloodstream.

Second, PTH works on the kidneys, making them excrete more phosphate and reabsorb more calcium from the filtered blood.

Third, PTH indirectly promotes the absorption of calcium, contained in the foods you eat, from your intestinal tract.

Low PTH levels, coupled with low calcium levels, usually indicate that the parathyroid glands have been damaged or removed. The consequences of low blood calcium are eventual convulsions, muscle spasms, even death.

Oversecretion of PTH, because of tumors or other proliferative changes of the glands, can lead to high calcium levels in the blood. This condition can eventually cause kidney stones, impaired kidney function, and serious loss of calcium from the skeleton. Fractures and other bone problems become common.

The test for PTH is usually done only after an initial screening test for calcium reveals levels outside the normal range. The parathyroid glands will usually be the logical place to look for the cause of the problem.

The major exception to these rules develops when kidney failure is present. The balance of phosphorus is upset, blood phosphorus becomes higher, calcium decreases in the blood, and the parathyroid glands react by releasing very large amounts of PTH. The bones lose more and more calcium unless the kidney condition improves or a special form of vitamin D is prescribed, 1,25 dihydroxy-$D_3$, a newly discovered product. This situation is called secondary hyperparathyroidism. A simple screening test for BUN reveals the inadequate function of the kidneys and explains the high PTH level in the face of normal or low blood calcium.

---

*Blood constituent: Human Growth Hormone (hGH)*
Normal range, males: Less than 6 nanograms per milliliter (ng/ml)
Normal range, females: Less than 10 nanograms per milliliter
Normal range, children: Up to 15 nanograms per milliliter

---

All of us have seen people who could be called dwarfs and others who can be considered to be giants; many have made their mark in show business or sports. Many others lead far less spectacular lives.

The purpose of this test is to determine if there is a hormonal basis to abnormal growth and development.

The causes of dwarfism or gigantism are primarily genetic, essentially all in the family. Only in the exceptional case is the growth hormone responsible. If the pituitary gland fails to secrete enough hGH in childhood, the person will remain undersized and develop dwarfism. Too much hGH, on the other hand, will cause the individual to become abnormally large and tall, reaching a height of up to seven or even eight feet.

During a youngster's growing years, the pituitary gland is responsible for providing enough growth hormone and for bringing about full sexual development at puberty. The timing of pubertal changes explains why some children are early developers, reaching their full height by the time they are fifteen. Others may do the bulk of their adolescent growing between eighteen to twenty-one. This is termed the adolescent growth spurt.

Other glands are also involved in the process of adult development. The thyroid, the pancreas, and the adrenal glands all produce hormones which interact with the effects of the growth hormone. It is a complicated effort, in which emotions can play an important role.

In adults, if the pituitary begins to produce excessive hGH after normal growth has been completed, body growth can resume in certain parts such as the hands, feet, lower jaw, and face. This condition is known as acromegaly and is caused by a benign pituitary tumor.

Acromegaly is often a slow-motion type of disease which remains unnoticed for years. People who have it eventually become aware that their hands, feet, nose, and tongue have enlarged and thickened. Most of the vital internal organs also increase in size, and a curvature of the spinal column may develop as its bones change in shape.

Acromegaly can cause a number of other glandular disturbances. There may be a sharp decrease in sexual activity, leading to impotence in men and loss of menstrual function in women. Diabetes may also develop. Despite an increase in the output of insulin, the excess hGH prevents the insulin from doing its work.

Too little growth hormone in adulthood is also harmful. While low hGH will not cause the person to shrink in stature, life may become miserable, with a weak, rundown feeling. The body will not be able to properly utilize fats as a source of energy. Kidney function may be impaired, and the bone marrow production of red blood cells may be below normal. Low blood sugar, with its mysterious symptoms, will usually be present.

In fact, whenever a patient has this assortment of abnormalities in the routine screening tests, the physician may well suspect that all the abnormalities could be the result of a single problem: low growth hormone. The doctor can double-check by ordering a follow-up hGH test, and if it is lower than expected for normal, additional confirmatory tests are indicated.

It is not uncommon for grownups to have low growth hormone at times, but they should be able to produce a fair amount of it on demand. The best way to provoke the pituitary into action is to drive the blood sugar down with an injection of insulin. Normal adults and children can raise the blood level of hGH to over 7 nanograms per milliliter, and most will achieve levels of 20 nanograms or more. An accurate diagnosis is essential, since children can be treated with injections of human growth hormone to stimulate growth. Adults do not need to grow and can be managed with a high-protein diet to combat weakness and low blood sugar. If insulin testing is not advisable, there are other "provocative" tests which use an injection of a pancreas hormone, glucagon, or an intravenous dosage of an amino acid, arginine, for this purpose.

One researcher has found that the arginine content of a generous serving of chopped liver is high enough to equal the dosage of an arginine test. This has not been put to practical use as a test, and the hGH levels would not remain high enough to restore growth. Perhaps the only point is that a bit of liver may not help but it certainly will not hurt a person with the problem of growth hormone deficiency.

When the diagnosis of acromegaly or of growth-hormone-caused gigantism is suspected, a screening sample for hGH is drawn, along with tests for glucose and phosphorus, which tend to go above normal in such cases. In order to prove that there is oversecretion of hGH, a glucose suppression test is done. The subject is at rest overnight, fasting after midnight, and is not allowed up even to the bathroom but must use a bedpan, since any exercise may raise the hGH level. The first blood samples are taken, and the person must then drink a flavored solution containing 100 grams of glucose, or over 3 ounces of sugar. This causes a major rise in the blood sugar level and a suppression of growth hormone production. In normal subjects, the hGH level drops below 5 nanograms per milliliter within one or two hours. The person with acromegaly continues to produce growth hormone and has hGH levels over 5 nanograms per milliliter at all times.

You may well ask, "Is all that testing necessary?" The answer is an unequivocal "Yes!" because curative treatments are available with one or more methods using radiation or surgery or a special drug.

---

*Blood constituent: Insulin*
Normal range, fasting: 4 to 24 microUnits per milliliter ($\mu$U/ml)

---

The purpose of this test is to determine problems with carbohydrate metabolism or with the pancreas in patients who may have diabetes or hypoglycemia; that is, too much or too little blood sugar.

Since its discovery and introduction into therapy by Drs. Frederick Grant Banting and Charles Herbert Best, insulin has become a household word. With millions of diabetics relying on daily doses of insulin or supportive medications for the control of their blood sugar levels, this hormone has come to be almost exclusively identified with glucose metabolism.

But insulin has other key metabolic functions. Insulin is instrumental in allowing certain amino acids to pass from the bloodstream into the body cells, where they are assembled into important proteins. Insulin also has the ability to convert and store excess energy from foods in the form of fatty tissues. And insulin is essential in enabling the body to utilize the phosphorus found in such foods as leafy vegetables, milk, and eggs.

How insulin does all of these things is still not completely known and remains the focus of considerable study to this day.

Insulin is manufactured in the pancreas gland, which is very sensitive to the level of glucose in the blood. As the concentration of sugar increases following a meal or a snack, insulin is secreted from the gland. Although the pancreas reacts most dramatically to sweets or sugar, these need not be included in what you eat. Any carbohydrate food, such as bread or potatoes, will soon be converted to glucose and require the pancreas to secrete more insulin.

Diabetes mellitus, or sugar diabetes, is the condition marked by a lack of sufficient insulin in the bloodstream. Damage to the pancreas through disease, genetic predisposition, and injury are the most common reasons for insulin insufficiency.

If a diabetic remains untreated—and there may be millions of unrecognized diabetics in the United States—the body will begin to suffer. The lack of insulin will make it impossible to convert enough carbohydrates into energy. The body will start using its proteins and fat reserves to sustain life, without being able to form the necessary amounts of new proteins or replenish its fat reserves. With these debilitating changes, body tissues and muscles will gradually waste away. The by-products of fatty tissue and muscle breakdown can build up to toxic levels in the blood, a condition known as ketosis or diabetic acidosis. The odor of one of these ketones, acetone (the same as the solvent used to remove nail polish), can appear on the breath, alerting the physician attending a patient in a coma.

Hypoglycemia, or too little sugar in the blood, may result from overproduction of insulin by the pancreas. Hypoglycemia could also be caused by inadequate secretion of the hormone cortisol by the adrenal glands. When blood sugar levels get too low, cortisol normally counteracts the effects of insulin until glucose levels return to normal.

The blood test for insulin is often done as a double check on the glucose tolerance test. The glucose test provides an indirect measure of insulin effects, while the insulin test gives the physician a direct measurement of how much insulin the pancreas gland is actually producing. In those cases of secondary diabetes caused by acromegaly, Cushing's disease, or the like, the blood levels of insulin may appear to be sufficient or actually higher than normal. The course of treatment will obviously need to be directed at the cause of this type of disturbance rather than at the diabetes, which is not due to true insulin deficiency.

Some authorities feel that insulin levels of hereditary diabetes mellitus patients reflect the stage of their disease. When the insulin becomes very low, additional treatment, perhaps insulin injections, may be needed. The newest test, glycohemoglobin, is being evaluated and is discussed in the section on glucose. It may reflect the exposure of red blood cells to elevated glucose levels over a three-month period. The exposed red blood cells form a derivative, glycosylated hemoglobin, which seems to be proportional to chronic glucose exposure during the lifetime of the red blood cell. This test could save having to do many blood or urine tests for glucose, and may improve treatment of the individual patient, since the "sugar coated" red cells may reveal the course of the diabetes and contribute to its diagnosis and control.

---

*Urine constituent: Total Estrogens*
Normal range, nonpregnant females: 4 to 105 micrograms per
    24-hour urine collection
Normal range, males: 4 to 25 micrograms per 24-hour urine
    collection

---

The purpose of this test is to help identify causes of female infertility, problems with sexual development in females, and adverse changes in males.

There is no single estrogen in the body. Estrogen is a collective designation for several female hormones with such names as estradiol, estrone, and estriol, with estradiol being the most potent. Estrogens are made primarily in the ovaries from cholesterol. But the adrenal glands in both sexes and the testicles in men are capable of estrogen production on a lesser scale.

Estrogens are very important in regulating the menstrual cycle, ensuring successful reproduction, and producing the typical feminine body characteristics of the mature woman. Although the normal measurement of estrogens is the total contained in a twenty-four hour urine specimen, many gynecologists first use vaginal cell smears to decide whether estrogens are below normal. In a doubtful case, the urine specimen is obtained to test for total estrogens. A blood sample can also be drawn to test for some of the specific components that make up estrogen.

The range for total estrogens in nonpregnant females is extremely changeable, with the result depending largely on when in the monthly cycle the urine specimen is collected. In pregnancy, the amount of estrogens can normally rise to hundreds of times the nonpregnant levels, sometimes reaching 40,000 micrograms per twenty-four-hour urine specimen.

Estrogen production in the ovaries is triggered at the beginning of puberty by FSH, or follicle stimulating hormone, produced by the pituitary gland. The estrogens transform the young girl into a woman, causing breast development and other changes in body contours, skeletal maturation, and growth of pubic hair.

The reasons for pituitary gland activation of the ovaries at puberty, by means of FSH, remain under study. Sometimes the pituitary turns on the FSH prematurely and a condition known as precocious puberty occurs. Parents who see their six-year-old suddenly take on the physical attributes of a woman become upset, more so than the child. Even tiny amounts of estrogens can be responsible for this situation. Early medical attention is needed to solve the problem and prescribe treatment before advanced development occurs. Such children will even have menstruation if the condition is allowed to progress. In fact, the earliest record-setting pregnancies have taken place in these fully developed children, who fail to understand the situation.

In diagnosing precocious puberty in females, it is important to determine if estradiol levels are high. If at the same time there is a low FSH result, it means that the pituitary gland is *not* at fault. The cause in such cases is usually a tumor of the ovary, which can be successfully removed—to the relief of the child and her parents.

During the first part of a normal menstrual cycle, estrogens act to create the most favorable conditions for conception in anticipation of the arrival of the male sperm. Estrogens cause development of the surface cells within the vaginal walls and thickening of the inner lining of the uterus. The glands in the cervix become more active and secrete increasing amounts of mucus, rather viscous in nature until ovulation, when it becomes watery.

When the egg is released from the ovary around the middle of the menstrual cycle, there is a decrease for a few days in the concentration of total estrogens, followed by a slight rise. Eventually, estrogen levels fall to an unmeasurable amount to signal the start of the following menstrual cycle.

What happens to total estrogens if pregnancy begins? After implantation of the fertilized egg and development of the placenta and fetus, the levels of estrogen increase dramatically. Large amounts of a second substance, progesterone, are produced by the corpus luteum, a structure that forms from the remnants of the ruptured follicle left behind in the ovary. Progesterone works with the estrogens to prepare the uterus to receive the fertilized egg. During pregnancy, progesterone also prevents contraction of the muscle tissues of the uterus and increases the development of the mammary glands for milk production. Should the physician suspect problems in any of these areas, a check of the blood level of progesterone would be made.

There are other sources of estrogens in the body, but far less than from the ovaries. The ovaries gradually shut down for the period of the pregnancy to prevent any release of more eggs that could lead to multiple births. The estrogen is then mainly produced in the placenta. In addition to providing nourishment to the fetus, the placenta manufactures estrogens from an adrenal hormone called dehydroepiandrosterone (DHEA), produced by the adrenal glands of the fetus. The estrogens promote the proper conditions within the mother to support growth of the developing baby.

Approximately five months after conception, the level of total estrogens again increases dramatically. Estriol, the major estrogen by-product which appears in the urine, is a useful indicator of whether the fetus is growing normally. Estriol makes up about 90 percent of the estrogens excreted during pregnancy.

If in the late months of pregnancy the level of estriol decreases markedly, then the possibility exists that the fetus is suffering some type of distress or may not be developing normally. The physician can use a series of blood or urine estriol tests to decide whether to deliver the baby early in order to save it.

Another cause of low estriol in the urine is a malfunction of the placenta. This problem is most common in diabetic mothers or women with kidney disease. The blood supply to the placenta ages prematurely and reaches old age before the fetus is mature. Sometimes the seven-month-old arteries in the placenta look like those of a seventy-year-old, and provide the fetus with diminishing supplies of oxygen, which could result in a stillbirth. Lower estrogen production is a sign of this condition and is likewise a warning to consider early induction of labor or a caesarian section to rescue the baby.

Adequate estradiol levels are known to be indispensable for successful pregnancy. During the late 1940s and 1950s it was a common practice to give synthetic estrogens to pregnant women who were having trouble carrying their babies to full term. One of these synthetic estrogens, called DES, for diethylstilbestrol, has been found to be associated with an increased incidence of cervical and vaginal abnormalities in the daughters of these women. This treatment has been abandoned, but as many as one million daughters may have been exposed. The young women who were brought into this world through the help of DES have been alerted to join a medical watch for reproductive-tract problems. There is a nationwide study called the DESAD (DES Adenosis) Project which assists in annual examinations.

Following a successful childbirth or a termination of pregnancy, the ovaries again produce estrogens. When the ovaries are no longer capable of estrogen production, menopause occurs. The supply of active follicles —the cells within the ovary that actually make estradiol—has become depleted, and there is no response despite increasing stimulation by the FSH hormone released from the pituitary. In fact, very high levels of FSH are typical of menopause because of this vain effort to prod the ovaries into action.

The sharp drop in estrogen levels during menopause contributes to the frequent hot flashes and irritability that many women experience at that time. Estrogen medication has been used to improve this condition, but is less favored nowadays due to concern about the possibility of side effects. Fortunately, even after menopause, some estrogens continue to be produced jointly by the adrenal glands and liver. This is usually enough to help women preserve their femininity after menopause and allow the troublesome symptoms to gradually improve.

In males, estrogens have the ability to counteract many of the effects of the male hormone, testosterone. Men with abnormally high levels of estrogens will assume many female characteristics. If estrogens are applied to the skin of males, the growth of body hair at that site will be reduced or stopped. The development of breast tissue in males can even be stimulated by the application of estrogens to the skin of the chest.

Spontaneous male breast development is occasionally observed. When a test reveals the presence of excess female hormones in the blood, the condition could be due to an adrenal or testicular tumor. But it could also be caused by a mistaken metabolism of hormones in the liver, as sometimes happens in the case of alcoholics. If the patient is suspected of concealing a history of alcohol abuse, a battery of liver function tests can provide an important clue. If confusion still exists as to the cause of the breast development, blood samples can be obtained by long plastic catheters inserted in major veins and moved close to various glands. A high estradiol level in the blood taken as it exits from a particular gland means that the gland harbors a tumor.

Estrogens are powerful substances—stimulators of biochemical reactions that can change important body functions. Much about their effects on our bodies still remains to be discovered. As a result the administration of estrogen medication has to be carefully watched by attentive and well-informed physicians.

---

*Blood constituent: Follicle Stimulating Hormone (FSH)*
Normal range, males: 5–20 milliInternational units per milliliter
   (mIU/ml)
Normal range, pre-menopausal females: 5–20 mIU/ml
Normal range, post-menopausal females: 50–200 mIU/ml

---

This test for follicle stimulating hormone, FSH, is very useful in cases of infertility. Taken together with selected endocrine tests, it can help to pinpoint some of the problems that tend to prevent conception.

FSH is released by the pituitary gland at the base of the brain, and derives its name from the action of this hormone on the follicles within the ovary. A follicle contains layers of cells that surround each egg in the ovaries. FSH is instrumental in developing these cells to create a complete follicle which resembles a nest for the egg.

FSH actually plays an important fertility role in both sexes. In males, FSH is essential for sperm production within the testicles.

The level of FSH in normal males remains fairly constant except for a slight pulsation normally detected at twenty-minute intervals. This pulsation represents the frequency with which the pituitary delivers FSH into the bloodstream.

Fertility problems in males are indicated when FSH levels are either too low or too high. If the levels are too low, the testes will not get the proper stimulation to be able to form sperm. Low FSH levels are usually an indication of pituitary gland problems or disorders in the hypothalamus portion of the brain.

If the levels of FSH are too high, it is an indication that the sperm-producing areas have become damaged or have failed to develop fully. The oversecretion of FSH is one of those typical responses of the body whereby it tries to activate a dormant or damaged system by extra doses of the specific substance that has a beneficial effect. Similar FSH elevations are seen in menopausal women or in women whose ovaries cannot respond to the FSH because of chromosomal abnormalities or damage from other causes.

The normal level of FSH in women seems to be inversely related to estrogen levels. By sensing the levels of estrogen in the bloodstream, the brain sends a message to the pituitary to release the proper amounts of FSH. Low estrogen levels appear to turn on the FSH output and high levels, to turn it off.

In women of childbearing age, estrogen levels change every day during the monthly cycle—and so do the levels of FSH. Here is a scenario for what may happen in a typical cycle.

After menstrual flow is completed and the next menstrual cycle begins, low estrogen levels call for an increasing supply of FSH from the pituitary. The plentiful FSH causes several egg-containing follicles in the ovary to start growing and maturing.

As this process continues, the cells within the most advanced follicle start to release estrogen. The gradual buildup of estrogen in the blood causes the hypothalamus to slow its production of gonadotropin-releasing factor, GnRH, and the pituitary gland has no choice but to trim its release of FSH, since GnRH is the only known stimulus to FSH secretion.

About the same time, the egg is released by the ovary in response to another chemical messenger, called luteinizing hormone, or LH. After the process of ovulation, the free egg migrates from the ovary to the entrance of the Fallopian tube and begins its descent to the uterus.

If fertilization does not take place, the egg will not implant in the uterus and the level of estrogen will start to decrease. This bottoming-out of the estrogen occurs near the beginning of the following menstruation and initiates a new cycle of FSH release from the pituitary for the subsequent development of the next follicle.

If fertilization does take place, estrogen levels increase dramatically and prevent further release of FSH. The next ovulation cycle is frozen, and the high estrogen levels prevail throughout the pregnancy.

---

*Blood constituent: Luteinizing Hormone (LH)*
Normal range, men: 5 to 20 milliInternational units per milliliter
    (mIU/ml)
Normal range, women: 8 to 28 milliInternational units per milliliter

Normal range, women at time of ovulation: 30 to 100
   milliInternational units per milliliter
Normal range, post-menopausal women: 50 to 200 milliInternational
   units per milliliter

---

The purpose of this test is to determine possible disease of the male
and female reproductive glands and of the pituitary gland.

LH has a great deal in common with FSH. Both are produced in
the pituitary gland, and both are involved in promoting certain functions
needed for fertility in men and women.

In men, LH is essential for the production of the principal male
hormone, testosterone, in the testes. Under normal circumstances, the
LH level in males is well sustained except for pulsations similar to those
of FSH, discussed in the preceding section.

In women of childbearing age, the level of LH increases dramatically as ovulation approaches. The pituitary gland pours out large quantities of the hormone to bring about the final development of the follicle
and the release of the egg.

The high levels of LH at this time have yet another function: to
convert the remnants of the ruptured follicle into the corpus luteum, a
structure capable of producing the hormone progesterone. Progesterone
is essential for successful implantation of a fertilized egg that has reached
the uterus.

Obviously, if LH levels at the time of ovulation are not sufficiently
high, conception will not be possible. The egg either will not be released
or will fail to be successfully implanted in the uterus. With respect to
men, inadequate levels of LH will result in low testosterone levels and
consequent impotence and sterility.

As with FSH, low LH levels may be caused by malfunctions of the
pituitary gland or the hypothalamus portion of the brain.

Abnormally high levels of LH are a sign that the reproductive
glands have been damaged by disease or removed by surgery. It is normal
for post-menopausal women to have similarly high LH levels when
castrated by total hysterectomy. Ovaries which have been spared such
surgery will cease their function at about the age of forty-eight. When
the ovaries become dormant, they no longer secrete enough estrogen for
menstruation to occur, and the low estrogen calls for a secondary rise
of LH as well as FSH to maximum levels.

When loss of male or female reproductive function is found, a low

LH indicates lack of hypothalamic–pituitary activity, and a high LH indicates that the reproductive glands have failed in their capacity to produce sex hormones.

---

*Blood constituent: Testosterone*
Normal range, male: 300 to 1200 nanograms per 100 milliliters
  (ng/100 ml)
Normal range, female: 0 to 100 nanograms per 100 milliliters

---

The purpose of this test is to diagnose male hormone deficiency in men or an excess of male hormone in women. The level of testosterone also provides a good indicator, in cases of male impotence, of whether it is related to physical deficiency or emotional disturbance.

Testosterone is the most important male hormone. It is responsible for such male characteristics as body hair, muscular development, and voice pitch—as well as body odor and acne in teenage boys.

Adequate testosterone is essential to a normal male sex drive. It is well known to physicians that the male with a deficiency of testosterone usually fails to register a complaint about his sex life, since he has lost the normal sexual desire. It is the wife who is more likely to notice this change in behavior. Also, a natural reluctance to reveal this personal problem often interferes with medical discovery and treatment.

Testosterone is primarily manufactured in the testes, with cholesterol playing an important role in the process. However, the adrenal glands of both sexes—and the ovaries of women in cases of certain disorders—can also indirectly make testosterone in lesser amounts with the help of the liver. A related compound, androstenedione, is released by the adrenal glands and ovaries. In turn, it is converted to testosterone in the liver cells and released again into the bloodstream.

In men castrated after puberty, this secondary testosterone production is occasionally sufficient to carry on near-normal male functions. A general decrease in such functions, even a loss of body hair, is more likely. But if castration or damage to the testes happens before puberty, normal sexual development will fail to take place altogether. Far greater amounts of testosterone are needed to initiate such development than to maintain it.

It may come as a shock to the male ego that testosterone holds no special sway over the female hormones, estrogens. In the proper dosage, estrogens can readily counter the effects of testosterone. In the case of prospective transsexuals—men wanting to become transformed into the physical shape of women—estrogens are administered to stimulate breast development and a feminine figure. In the poultry industry, female hormones used to be administered to male birds to produce capons with the plump, full-breasted shape of hens.

Women occasionally have problems with elevated levels of testosterone. They develop facial hair, the voice deepens, and menstruation becomes irregular. In more advanced stages, a full beard can form, the clitoris becomes enlarged, and the rounded female form may take on some of the muscular characteristics of men. This condition is usually caused by improper functioning of the ovaries, adrenal glands, or liver due to tumors or enzymatic defects. Once the delicate balance between estrogens and testosterone is brought back to normal, the symptoms will gradually disappear. Vigorous hair follicles may require electrolysis to eliminate the last traces of facial hair.

# 9
# Sex-Related Testing

As age-old taboos concerning human sexuality are replaced by open curiosity, medical research in this field is providing us with more answers and alternative courses of action. It could perhaps be said that the sexual revolution is being matched by a laboratory testing revolution.

Some of the tests described in this chapter are only for women and others are only for men. What all the tests have in common is that they are related to human sexual and reproductive functions.

We should not forget, despite all the present-day emphasis on the pleasures of sex, that the primary biological function of sex is procreation. Although the survival of humanity no longer depends on a sustained high birth rate, the process of creating a life can be one of the most important of all events for us on a personal level.

The first part of the chapter is devoted to tests related to various aspects of conception and the different ways of helping to bring it to a successful conclusion. The remaining tests are related to sexual health and hygiene, and might very well save somebody from a great deal of suffering and possibly very serious complications.

## Fertility/Female

In today's world, most people are concerned with spacing or preventing conception. Yet for about 10 percent of married women, the opposite is the case. They experience the anxiety of being unable to conceive and would do anything within reason to reach that goal.

Although many of the causes of infertility remain obscure, some are related to an imbalance of various female hormones. These imbalances can be evaluated and measured, and corrective action can frequently be taken to make natural motherhood possible.

As in other disorders, the various tests which may help reverse infertility begin with a general examination. The first step involves a careful investigation of the reproductive organs. If there are no mechanical difficulties such as blocked Fallopian tubes or large fibroid tumors in the uterus, then the general health of the patient is studied in greater detail. The woman's emotional state and physical condition are considered as potential clues, and the possibility of glandular disorders is examined.

One of the test groups the doctor is likely to order is a check for thyroid function. Even if the woman is unaware of any symptoms, a subnormal level of thyroid hormone can prevent conception. The normal ranges for thyroid tests are rather broad. In the individual case, a subtle deficiency capable of preventing conception could exist with seemingly normal results. Some doctors will even prescribe a course of thyroid hormone for about three months to eliminate or confirm that possibility.

If the doctor sees any signs of male-hormone action such as extra hair on the woman's face, breasts, or lower abdomen, the problem could be caused by an excess of male hormones. A twenty-four-hour urine collection would be tested for 17-ketosteroids (break down products of male hormones). A blood sample would be drawn to check for any excess amounts of testosterone and androstenedione (principal male hormones in the bloodstream).

Before any treatment involving fertility drugs can be considered, the doctor will need to learn more about the function of the ovaries. If the ovaries are enlarged and rough-surfaced due to cyst formation, the patient might be treated with a mild fertility drug designed to restore ovulation. If the problem persists, a wedge resection operation to trim the ovaries can often restore normal function and a rapid return to fertility. Pregnancy usually occurs within the first three months after surgery, much to the delight and surprise of the would-be parents.

If the menstrual cycle is erratic, a fertility drug is available to regulate the cycle and induce ovulation at a predictable time. But if the cycle is apparently normal, then more hormone tests are needed.

Among those substances tested will be the pituitary hormones, FSH and LH. They are instrumental in making the ovaries develop their eggs and release them. Because of improper levels, the action of these hormones may not be synchronized properly to cause the release of a mature egg so that conception can take place. In that case, menstrual periods would still occur but without ovulation.

FSH levels also affect the levels of estrogens in the body. If FSH levels are not high enough, the amount of estrogens made by the ovaries may not be sufficient to prepare the lining of the uterus for receiving the fertilized egg. When the gynecological examination and vaginal-smear cytology test support this possibility, the doctor will check the estrogen level by ordering a blood test for estradiol, the main component of estrogens in the body.

Another test the doctor may order is for progesterone. This hormone is secreted by the corpus luteum left behind after ovulation where the egg had developed in the ovary. If the woman does not have enough progesterone, the lining of the uterus will not develop sufficiently for successful implantation of a fertilized egg.

During fetal development, progesterone is also necessary to prevent contractions of the muscles of the uterus—which could result in premature labor. In early pregnancy, not enough progesterone could result in a spontaneous abortion.

It is obvious that the factors relating to a woman's fertility are numerous and complex. Sometimes it helps to check on the entire reproductive system by taking a small snip of tissue from the lining of the uterus toward the end of the monthly cycle. The tissue is studied under a microscope for signs of estrogen and progesterone action on the cells.

This simple and almost painless test can direct the gynecologist to the central problems that need attention. In rare cases, an inadequate lining is caused by infection or other injuries leading to scar formation. Considerable time and effort are saved by early diagnosis. If there is a need for this type of test, it will be suggested after the preliminary examinations have been done.

The latest test for helping correct female infertility measures the prolactin hormone in the blood. Secreted by the pituitary gland, this hormone promotes milk production and prevents ovulation. Even primitive people took advantage of this form of birth control by prolonging breast-feeding. When prolactin levels are high, FSH and LH levels remain low and menstrual periods come to a halt. This is natural during the breast-feeding period. But what if prolactin levels are high in a person who is not breast-feeding or who has never even been pregnant?

The first clue is a congested sensation in the breasts or even leakage of liquid into the clothing. During an examination, the doctor will be able to bring milk to the nipples by gently massaging the breasts. The condition may be due to certain tranquilizer drugs which can raise prolactin levels and cause milk formation. If no drugs are involved, then the condition is probably due to a small, benign growth of cells within the pituitary gland. Even if pregnancy were possible, it should be avoided unless the condition is corrected. Untreated tumors have been known to enlarge during pregnancy.

Once corrected—either through radiation therapy or a new surgical procedure in which the tumor is removed through the nasal cavity—pregnancy can occur. If any extra prolactin is still being secreted, it can usually be stopped by a new medication which works within weeks once the proper dosage is achieved.

Prolactin tests are essential for monitoring the effects of treatment. Many doctors are still unfamiliar with both the condition and the test, since most medical textbooks have not yet been updated to reflect this knowledge. Prolactin test results are usually slow in returning. This is because laboratories often save such uncommon samples for several days until they have a sufficient number to process. Within the next few years, this test and its relation to infertility will become more commonplace, and results will be available very quickly.

## Fertility/Male

In a childless marriage, the woman has traditionally been considered to be "at fault." Yet up to 50 percent of infertile marriages may well be due to the male partner's inability to fertilize his mate.

As with any investigation for abnormal conditions within the body, the evaluation of male infertility should begin with a careful physical examination and history of personal habits. The examination should focus not only on the male genital organs but on the person's physical condition in general. Among the relevant personal habits might be alcohol usage, exposure to radiation, emotional stress, smoking, and exercise.

The physician would take special note as to how the person's glandular systems are functioning. The thyroid, pituitary, and adrenal glands work closely with the testes to create the right conditions for male fertility. The physician might order a number of specific hormonal tests, such as the principal male hormone, testosterone, to ensure that the levels are within normal ranges.

Some genetic testing might also be indicated. These particular tests can be expensive, costing up to a hundred dollars each. The doctor would usually want to have good reason to order a chromosome analysis, such as signs of small testes or enlarged breasts, which are typical of some genetic abnormalities.

In the normal male, the Y chromosome, which determines the genetic male, is paired with an X chromosome, as XY. If because of an inborn defect the male has XXY instead of the normal XY, he has Klinefelter's syndrome—and is very likely to be infertile. Even if the male has XYY sex chromosomes, he may still be sterile, despite the presence of a double amount of male genetic material. It seems to be important to have the balanced pair of one X and one Y chromosome to function normally.

Perhaps the most familiar phase of fertility testing is the semen examination. Even though it takes only one sperm cell to fertilize the egg, the sperm cells contained in semen should be of sufficient numbers, be properly shaped, and be able to swim vigorously to provide the best chances of fertilization. They have a long way to travel to fertilize the egg. Many of the millions contained in a single ejaculation will fail to reach their target. But the more sperm cells there are and the healthier they are, the better the chances that one of them will find and fertilize the egg.

To evaluate semen, care must be taken in collecting it. Many men are reluctant to be tested, since it usually requires that they masturbate or withdraw before completion of orgasm in order to collect the specimen. The ejaculated semen should be collected in a clean glass jar or in a special mylar plastic condom that has no spermicide gel or chemical coating. The specimen must be kept warm and brought promptly to the laboratory. If more than three hours elapse after collection, the sperm cells may change in appearance or lose their ability to move, thus giving misleading results.

The usual volume of semen is one-half to one full teaspoon of fluid, with sperm cells swimming within the fluid in all directions. More seminal fluid does not necessarily mean more sperm cells. Quite the opposite may be the case. After special preparation of the sample, the laboratory technician will examine the semen under a microscope to get the essential data on the number of sperm cells, their ability to move, and their shape.

The normal range for the number of sperm cells varies between 60 and 150 million per milliliter of semen. If the total number is less than 25 million per milliliter, the count is considered to be subnormal. That does not mean that anyone with a lower count will not be able to father a child; only that the chances will be significantly reduced.

As for motility, or the ability of the sperm cells to move in the fluid, normal semen contains about 75 percent or more sperm cells that show definite motility. If 50 to 60 percent are non-motile, then the semen is considered abnormal. Fatherhood, under these conditions, is again not impossible but more uncertain.

Deformities in the shapes of the sperm cells can show up as sperm with excessively small or excessively large "heads"; as single heads with two "tails," or single tails with two heads; or as constricted heads or even heads that are grossly misshapen. In normal semen, less than 30 percent of the sperm cells are deformed. If a majority of the sperm cells are deformed, then conception is less probable.

Any abnormal findings should be confirmed with additional fresh specimens. Each specimen should be collected after at least three days' abstinence from coitus. Or the time interval for the male's customary sexual activity may be designated for collection of the semen. If the male is sexually active once a month or less often, the physician may require a specimen much sooner. The reason is that a prolonged time period between coitus may cause the sperm cells stored in the testes to become abnormal in their shape and ability to move.

If the sperm concentration is abnormally low, the physician may order additional hormone tests. These may include tests for the pituitary hormone, FSH, which stimulates the production of sperm cells, and LH, which promotes the production of the male hormone, testosterone, in the testes.

Semen evaluation is also used for an opposite purpose. For men who have undergone a vasectomy, this test lets them know when they can engage in intercourse without any further chance of impregnating their mate. To confirm that the operation is complete, there should be no sperm cells in the semen in an evaluation performed three months after the vasectomy.

As for impotency problems in male infertility, these are usually treated as emotional rather than physical, provided that there is a sufficient level of the male hormone testosterone and no major disease such as diabetes mellitus or cirrhosis of the liver.

## Pregnancy Testing

Depending on the situation, the results of this test may be awaited with either joyful anticipation or subdued trepidation. It is the only test where a positive finding in a woman with a "missed" or "delayed" menstrual period does not augur some insidious disease but the creation of life itself.

Although the techniques of pregnancy testing have changed considerably over the years, they are all based on the same principle: detection of a hormone called chorionic gonadotropin, or HCG, released by the uterus as soon as membranes begin to develop to nourish the fetus. About two weeks following conception, the level of HCG begins to rise in the blood and spills over into the urine.

A new and highly sensitive blood test now removes virtually all of the traditional waiting and uncertainty from pregnancy testing. Using radioactively labeled chemicals, this test can provide an accurate measure of HCG in the blood sample within ten to fourteen days after conception. Often the verdict is in even before the woman would ordinarily have her next period.

This new blood test is also useful in monitoring the early stages of pregnancy. By accurately measuring the amounts of HCG in the blood at periodic intervals, the doctor has another indicator as to whether the pregnancy is progressing normally.

Although the new HCG blood test is probably going to be increasingly used in the future to determine pregnancy, most of the pregnancy testing today still relies on detecting HCG in urine. Most laboratories and doctors are geared for the urine test, and most home testing kits are based on the same principles. Besides, the HCG blood test is about twice as expensive as the urine test.

The problem with the urine test is the difficulty of being able to detect the minute quantities of HCG early enough. Some years ago, this used to be known as the rabbit test because the only way of checking for HCG was to inject the urine sample into a female rabbit. The animal was then killed and its ovaries checked for the characteristic changes that would be brought about by the presence of HCG.

Today the techniques for detecting HCG in the urine are far more refined, and no animal need be sacrificed. Yet it still takes about six weeks after the time of supposed conception before a reasonably certain answer can be given, one way or the other.

In the meantime, there may be various physical signs raising the possibility of pregnancy. The normal menstrual period will not have occurred, the breasts will usually be tender and swollen, and there may be morning sickness. A pelvic examination would reveal a softening and magenta coloration of the cervix. Should the examination take place four or five weeks after conception, the uterus and cervix may be detectably enlarged, with perhaps more frequent urination as the enlarged uterus begins to press against the bladder. At this point, a urine specimen would usually contain enough HCG to be measurable.

Different laboratories use techniques of different sensitivity for detecting HCG in the urine. The objective is to be able to make a definite determination at the earliest possible time with the greatest degree of accuracy. It is really a trade-off. If the technique is overly sensitive, designed to detect HCG as early as possible, there may be a higher number of false positives—indicating pregnancies when they do not exist. If the test is not one of the extremely sensitive types, it may give more false negative results—failing to detect pregnancies, especially in the first few weeks. For the most part, laboratory tests of HCG have been designed to provide about 95 percent accuracy at five to six weeks following conception. But there are individual differences. One woman may have sufficient HCG in her urine to be accurately detected in the fifth week of pregnancy; another woman may not have detectable HCG until at least six or seven weeks. For some people, that may seem like an interminable wait.

Other factors can also give false positive or false negative results. If the urine is too dilute or if the specimen has been left standing too long at room temperature, the result can be a false negative. Usually an early-morning specimen analyzed immediately will overcome these problems.

False positive pregnancy tests can occur with some detection methods if there is too much protein or too many blood cells in the urine. Detergents in the collection cup as well as the use of certain drugs, such as phenothiazine in tranquilizers, can sound a false alarm.

The home pregnancy tests that have been developed and marketed as a do-it-yourself alternative are based on methods similar to those used in laboratories. The same factors which can cause a false positive or false negative result in a laboratory affect the home tests—and even more so. In laboratories, there is a constant quality control system which uses known positive and negative samples. The technicians are highly experienced in the procedure, and their chemicals and equipment are constantly being double-checked. The home pregnancy tests obviously are not infallible and should be interpreted with professional assistance if confirmation is needed.

## Amniocentesis

The purpose of amniocentesis is to check the fetus for possible genetically related diseases and other disorders so that corrective action can be taken. An incidental benefit of this test is that the parents can find out the sex of their expected child, even months in advance of birth.

Amniocentesis derives its name from the amniotic fluid which bathes and protects the developing fetus in the mother's womb. As with blood and urine, this fluid can be removed and tested for various constituents which foretell certain information about the unborn baby.

To obtain a sample of amniotic fluid, a sterilized needle is inserted, under local anesthesia, through the woman's abdomen into the womb. A small amount of the fluid is removed by means of a syringe for analysis by special laboratory techniques. Since amniotic fluid is formed by the urinary tract of the fetus and surrounds the baby within the womb, the sample contains chemical by-products and surface cells from the fetus.

Perfected over the past twenty-five years, the procedure is relatively painless and is considered to carry few risks for either mother or fetus. However, amniocentesis should never be done just to satisfy the curiosity of the parents about the sex of their future child. The procedure is warranted only in situations where there is suspicion about the possibility of abnormal conditions in the fetus such as mongolism, which is more prevalent after a maternal age of thirty-five.

If there is a history of family-related disorders, fetal cells from the amniotic fluid can be cultured and analyzed for their genetic makeup. Through a process called karyotyping, the number and kinds of normal and abnormal chromosomes are determined. Karyotyping can identify such genetically related problems as Down's syndrome, or mongolism, with a triple twenty-first chromosome; Klinefelter's syndrome, with an extra female X chromosome added to the male XY group; and Turner's syndrome, in which one of the two female X chromosomes is absent. There is evidence that sickle cell anemia, which already affects over 70,000 people in the United States, may also be detected in fetal cells obtained from amniotic fluid.

If there is a suspicion that the developing fetus is suffering from hemolytic anemia as a result of the mother's antibodies attacking and destroying the baby's red blood cells, the analysis of amniotic fluid may reveal the presence of bilirubin. Bilirubin elevations may signify destruction of red blood cells. If bilirubin elevations are found to be significant, then the physician will need to consider early delivery to save the fetus.

A special test on the amniotic fluid can assess the development of the baby's lungs by measuring two chemicals called lecithin and sphingomyelin. Before the thirty-fifth week of pregnancy, these materials are released by the developing lungs in about equal quantities. In the thirty-fifth week, the amount of lecithin released normally jumps to about four times the concentration of sphingomyelin. As the lungs continue to develop, even more lecithin is released. If the physician has to induce a premature birth, the ability of the fetus to breathe on its own has to be determined. An indicator of fetal lung capacity is obtained with this lecithin/sphingomyelin test on amniotic fluid, the "L-S ratio" test.

Not only is amniocentesis saving countless lives, it frequently spares prospective parents needless worry. People are becoming increasingly aware of what can cause deformities in the newborn. The list includes not only genetic disorders such as Tay-Sachs disease, but exposure to noxious chemicals or toxic contaminants; viral diseases such as German measles or herpes; motherhood after the age of thirty-five; or even having a couple of drinks a day or smoking a daily pack of cigarettes during pregnancy. The test results usually either put an end to parental concern or lead to remedial steps, which will depend on the stage of fetal development.

Already popular, amniocentesis is likely to become increasingly used in the future, and new methods are being constantly developed to gain still more specialized information from the amniotic fluid about the condition of the fetus.

## Rubella Test

This could be a very important test for women planning to have children. Some states require the rubella test before issuing a marriage license; other states recommend it.

Rubella is the name of the virus that causes German measles. The purpose of the test is to find out whether the individual has been previously exposed to the disease and has obtained lasting immunity to it. If the prospective mother had no prior exposure, German measles can be a cause of tremendous concern. The disease can result in severe damage to the fetus, especially if it strikes in the early stages of pregnancy.

The rubella test measures the level of antibodies to this virus. If the level is low or negative, then the person is still susceptible to the infection. In such a case, the physician may advise the woman planning on motherhood to be vaccinated against rubella well ahead of time and have one less thing to worry about during her pregnancy.

Some women may find that they actually have enough antibodies against the virus to give them immunity, even though they are not aware that they ever had the disease. This is because they might have built up the antibodies during a casual exposure that did not produce any noticeable symptoms. The test will show whether these antibodies would be sufficient to protect the unborn baby during any possible future exposure of the mother to rubella.

## Pap Test

Named after its developer, Dr. George Papanicolaou, the Pap test is used to screen women for cervical cancer. The test permits early detection of the cancer and provides the best chance to overcome the consequences of this disease.

Many doctors do a Pap test as a matter of routine for women undergoing a general physical or annual gynecological examination. The incidence of cervical cancer in the United States is approximately nine per 100,000 per year. Certain groups have a higher incidence than others. Women who have a long history of sexual activity with multiple partners and women whose male partners are uncircumcised are among those with higher rates. The greatest incidence of cervical cancer is among women between twenty-one and thirty-five years of age.

The Pap test may also detect cancers arising within the womb, provided that a sufficient number of endometrial cells lining the uterus have been shed through the cervical opening into the vagina.

In taking a specimen for a Pap test, the physician gently scrapes the entrance to the cervix with a wood spatula and smears the scraped cells on a glass slide. A second smear is usually taken with a pipette from the vaginal liquid pool located in the space behind the neck of the cervix.

If you have ever had a Pap test, you may have seen an aerosol can of hair spray handily located nearby. It is certainly *not* used to spray the genital region to tidy up after an examination—but to cover the cells on the glass slide and protect them before they are analyzed. Another method involves a quick immersion of the slides into a preservative solvent solution.

In the laboratory, the collected cells are stained with special dyes to highlight the nucleus and other cellular materials. The results are evaluated by cytotechnologists, who specialize in detecting cancers from areas that cannot be easily examined directly. They evaluate whether the cells removed from the genital canal are normal or show any abnormal changes. Suspicious readings are reviewed carefully by the pathologist in charge, who is a physician trained to analyze cellular changes that may signal disease.

From the size, shape, and intensity of the staining, the cells are categorized into normal and abnormal findings. The changes often are subtle and only a few cells on the glass slides may show abnormal characteristics. But it takes only one abnormal cell to indicate a possible cause for concern.

The changes in cellular characteristics vary over a range of possibilities before a definite cancerous condition can be diagnosed. A normal finding is reported as a class 1 or "negative" result.

If there is inflammation for whatever reason, the results can be reported as a class 2a. A class 2b, the next higher grade, represents slight to moderate changes which indicate more abnormal characteristics of the cells.

Class 3 is moderate to severe dysplasia, or abnormal cellular changes, which may require a follow-up colposcopy examination by the physician. Colposcopy makes use of a microscope-like device to view the cervix and look for any white, abnormal patches of surface tissue around the opening of the cervix. Biopsy specimens of these patches may be taken for detailed pathological examination.

Class 4 and class 5 designations refer to more progressive changes in the cervical cells, with an increased likelihood that the changes are cancerous. A biopsy will have to be taken of the cervix for definite confirmation of cervical cancer through the use of histologic techniques. A class 5 is the highest result for the Pap smear, signifying that there is a very high probability of cervical cancer.

The numerical designation system is gradually being replaced by an identification of the type of abnormal cellular changes observed in a Pap specimen. Instead of a number, the Pap test result will be an actual description of the characteristics of the cells. The physician will base any follow-up procedures on the nature and severity of the changes in the cells.

Once cervical cancer is diagnosed from biopsied specimens, the treatment can vary. It can include anything from a complete hysterectomy to merely freezing the cells of the abnormal area by a process called cryosurgery. The freezing process causes the abnormal cells—and also many normal cells—in the cervical tissue to die and be eventually shed. If the new cells replacing those that have been removed are normal, the cryosurgery was successful in removing the cancer.

Cancer within the uterus lining, which also can be detected by the Pap test, usually occurs in women who are over the age of fifty and probably past menopause. Any unusual pain, bleeding, or discharge from the uterus of post-menopausal women should be investigated by a scraping of the cervical area and also by taking a biopsy from inside the womb. The cervical smear may contain some of the endometrial cells which indicate the state of health within the uterus. These cells are stained with the same or similar dyes as for cervical cells, and the grading of the results is also similar. A review by a pathologist will confirm or eliminate the possibility of an intrauterine tumor.

Any Pap test which shows slight to moderate changes in the cells lining the inner cervix or uterus should be repeated by the physician within a few months. Whatever changes are observed may be crucial to the diagnosis. It is not unusual to see negative findings on a subsequent smear. But these will have to be confirmed by still another smear a few months later.

The accuracy of determining cervical cancer from scrapings taken from the vicinity of the cervix is about 95 percent. With similar techniques, the accuracy for finding cancer within the uterus lining—or endometrial cancer—is about 60 percent. It is hoped that new methods will be developed to find the other 40 percent which at present elude the Pap test.

## Prostatic Acid Phosphatase Test (Male PAP)

The main purpose of this test is to help in the early detection of tumors or cancers affecting the prostate gland. Often known as the male PAP test, this test might in the future be used as widely to screen men for prostate cancers as the female counterpart test is used for cervical cancers.

The test is a very simple one, since it involves measuring the level of prostatic acid phosphatase in a blood sample. Acid phosphatase is a type of enzyme which is found in certain tissues of both males and females, but one such enzyme is present in relatively large quantities in the male prostate gland.

A normal level of the enzyme is not always a guarantee that there is no cancer in the prostate gland. Also, an elevated level may have been caused by prostate massage, prostate examination, or by the drug clofibrate. Otherwise, an elevated level is usually an indication of the possibility of cancer of the prostate.

There is another sort of test for prostatic acid phosphatase for a totally different purpose; namely, to obtain evidence of intercourse when rape has taken place. Since prostatic acid phosphatase appears in seminal fluid, the victim's vaginal canal is washed with a solution, after which it is collected and sent to the laboratory. Checking for prostatic acid phosphatase is superior to merely testing for the presence of sperm, since some rapists could have abnormal gland function and produce no sperm. Vasectomy would have the same effect. Moreover, prostatic acid phosphatase will show up seventy-two hours after ejaculation, whereas sperm will rarely last more than a day or two.

## Syphilis Test

The test for syphilis remains a prerequisite for a marriage license in most states. It is also part of the admission testing for most hospital patients. To the pregnant mother, syphilis is a major concern since it can cause serious abnormalities in the fetus or spontaneous abortion. Traditionally known as the Wasserman, the test for syphilis now goes under a half-dozen different names, reflecting the different techniques utilized. The results are reported as either positive or negative.

Syphilis is an infection with the organism *Treponema pallidum,* regardless of the site. It is one of the few venereal diseases which can be transmitted by kissing. But most often, the primary infection site is the sexual organs.

In females, the first signs of syphilis may be difficult to detect. A slow-healing sore on the genitalia may be visible, but is just as likely to be hidden within the vagina or on the cervix. Antibodies formed against the invading organism can be detected through blood tests about three to four weeks following infection.

In males, the primary stage of the disease is usually more evident. If the penis is the site of the infection, a clearly visible sore called a chancre will form within about ten days after contact. Using a "darkfield" illumination under a microscope, a scraping from the sore will reveal the spiral-shaped organisms that cause the disease.

In the secondary stage, about forty-five to ninety days after exposure, lesions may appear on the skin of the body or inside the mouth. But these too may heal spontaneously before medical attention is sought.

The third and often terminal stage can develop years later, causing disease of the nervous system, internal organs, and blood vessels. The symptoms at this point may mimic a variety of other serious diseases. For this reason, syphilis has been called the great impostor. A specific test is the only way to make the correct diagnosis.

With early detection, syphilis can be treated with penicillin or other antibiotics to prevent serious and often fatal consequences.

In testing for syphilis, false positive tests may occur. More specific testing methods will then be employed to avoid emotional distress and unnecessary treatment. Thus, in the absence of other obvious symptoms or a known history of venereal infection, a positive result will not be taken as a final answer.

## Gonorrhea Test

In women, the test for gonorrhea through special culturing techniques is sometimes the only way to detect this disease. In men, the symptoms are usually more easily detected by a smear of the penile discharge.

The typical symptoms of gonorrhea in men include inflammation of the urinary or genital tract and a discharge of pus and mucus from the penis. In women, there may only be a sense of irritation in the pelvic region, which is often mistaken for intestinal pains. In many women, there are no symptoms at all, and the condition may remain undiagnosed until peritonitis develops and requires emergency surgery.

Untreated gonorrhea in women may lead to permanent infertility because of closure of the Fallopian tubes, which allow the egg to migrate to the uterus. Scar tissue can form in and around these delicate tubes to cause complete blockage, unless surgery is able to correct it. An untreated case could progress to such a stage that a total hysterectomy might have to be performed. In men, untreated gonorrhea may spread to the prostate gland, creating problems for years to come.

Gonorrhea is transmitted only by direct sexual contact, since the infecting organism, *Neisseria gonorrheae,* does not survive for long when exposed to the oxygen in the air. Consequently, the culture plates must be incubated under a carbon dioxide atmosphere in special cabinets.

## Herpes Test

Infection by the herpes virus in the sexual organs is rapidly becoming one of the most common of all venereal diseases. One reason for its high incidence is that there is as yet no permanent cure and the disease may recur spontaneously without reinfection by sexual contact.

There are two distinct types of herpes viruses which have been identified. Type 1 affects adults and children only above the waist, and type 2, usually only adults below the waist. Type 1 is not considered to be in any way a venereal disease. The most common and noticeable sign of type 1 herpes infection is the cold sore at the corner of the mouth. But this virus can also affect other parts of the face, the eyes, and the skin above the waist, causing an eczema-like reaction.

In its severest form, type 1 herpes can make its way into brain tissue, and cause encephalitis and neurologic disturbances which can sometimes be fatal. The special blood test for herpes is the only test to identify that very serious form of the disease, other than a biopsy of affected tissue.

Type 2 herpes can also result in serious problems, especially for women. This type of herpes may infect the vagina and cervix, where it may not even be noticed. But often there will be a vaginal discharge, genital pain, or bleeding after intercourse. There may also be a feeling of malaise a few days before the discharge or pain.

In men, the symptoms are more obvious. There is usually an itchy rash with tiny blisters, which eventually break and form scabs. Except for the location, on the penis, the signs of herpes 2 infection are similar to those of cold sores on the face.

Herpes 2 is initially transmitted by sexual intercourse. With abstinence from intercourse, the symptoms will usually clear up within two weeks. Subsequent infections, however, may be triggered by emotional disturbances, onset of the menstrual period, a generally rundown condition, or many as yet unidentified factors that seem to vary from individual to individual. Some people may get the infection once, never to be bothered by it again; others will scarcely recover from one infection when the next one begins. A permanent cure by specific medication is hoped for in the near future.

In addition to causing the unpleasantness of repeated herpes 2 infections, this virus is being considered as a possible factor in cervical cancer, especially in younger women.

In pregnant women, herpes 2 virus can threaten the well-being of the fetus. Should the prospective mother have a spontaneous flare-up of a herpes 2 infection during the early months of pregnancy, the effect on the fetus could be similar to that of German measles, i.e., a risk of birth defects. Should the infection occur when delivery is about to take place, there would be a danger of infecting the baby during its passage through the birth canal. Surgical intervention by caesarian section may be the only way to avoid this risk.

Besides the special blood test used to screen for the presence of herpes 2, a cytology Pap smear is another way of identifying the active form of the disease.

## *Nonvenereal Vaginitis Test*

Nonvenereal vaginal infections are far more common than venereal ones, and often, far more difficult to cure. Although not life-threatening or serious in themselves, such infections can sometimes put an indefinite damper on a couple's sexual life, with serious emotional consequences.

Among the most common nonvenereal vaginal infections are moniliasis, caused by the organism *Candida albicans;* trichomoniasis, caused by a tiny, fast-moving creature in the protozoa category; and another form of vaginitis caused by a bacteria called *Hemophilus vaginalis.*

All three conditions have similar symptoms of excessive discharge and various degrees of vaginal discomfort. Since the cause of each of these conditions is a different type of organism, the treatment in each case is also different. It is therefore most important to diagnose properly the exact nature of the infection. Sometimes two or even three of these infections can be present at the same time.

To identify the organisms causing the problem, smears taken from the vaginal canal must be submitted to the laboratory for analysis. The procedure in collecting and preserving the smears and then identifying them in the laboratory will be slightly different in each case. The diagnostic experience of the physician is an important factor in deciding what the suspicious organism may be so that the proper culturing techniques can be employed.

Sometimes the organism may be harbored in the urethra or prostate gland of the man. Although he may have no symptoms, he will continue to reinfect his partner unless he too is treated. This is especially true in the case of trichomoniasis, for which there is now a highly effective drug for curing both partners. If there is any suspicion that the male partner may indeed be the carrier, a smear of prostatic fluid should be cultured to resolve the situation.

This condition has often been called a Ping-Pong type of infection because of the to-and-fro transfer of the infection. But unlike in the game, when this happens both partners are losers.

# 10
# Testing Your Vitamin Levels

Vitamins are at the center of one of the more heated controversies of our time. Millions of people believe that vitamins, if taken in sufficient doses, can cure or prevent virtually every ailment under the sun. Other people consider this claim to be nothing but an advertising ploy, foisted on the public by vitamin manufacturers interested in profits.

That vitamins are essential to life, no one can dispute. Vitamins are organic chemicals which your body, for the most part, cannot manufacture. They must be derived almost entirely from the food you eat or from supplements. The intricate process called life requires vitamins for cell growth, metabolic reactions, and the normal functioning of tissues and nerves.

Knowledge of vitamins goes as far back as 2,400 years ago when Hippocrates advised his patients with defective night vision to eat liver. What they lacked was vitamin A. The British put their intuition about vitamins to work in the 1800s when they served limes to their sailors on long voyages in order to prevent scurvy. What these sailors (who acquired the name "limeys") were getting was vitamin C. And in the first part of this century, vitamin D was first added to our milk supply to prevent the disease known as rickets.

Vitamins are often divided into two general categories: those that are readily soluble in water, and those that are soluble in fat. The water-soluble vitamins consist of the B-complex group and vitamin C. These are rapidly eliminated in the urine, and must be supplied on a daily basis. Vitamins A, D, E, and K are dissolved by fats and tend to get stored in body tissues when taken in excess. It is far more common for people to suffer from an overdose of these vitamins than of the water-soluble type.

The controversy today concerns the quantities of vitamins that we should be getting. Vitamin advocates admit that the recommended daily requirements may indeed be enough to prevent such damaging diseases as scurvy and rickets. But they also maintain that we need far greater than the recommended quantities as a protection against our polluted environment, and still greater quantities if we are to derive some of their reputed therapeutic effects. The argument as to whether massive doses of vitamin C, for example, are effective against the common cold and other infections continues unresolved, with eminent proponents on both sides of the issue.

The last word on vitamins is not yet in. Since the establishment of the minimum daily requirements many decades ago, research in this area has lagged until the recent upsurge. It is a very complex field. What is essential for some animal species may not be needed by the human race. And there may well be a major difference between you and your neighbor as to how much of a particular vitamin you need for a healthy life.

Little wonder, then, that many people are beginning to ask their doctors about vitamins; how much to take, which ones, in what form, on what occasions? Some people would even like to know whether the vitamin levels in their bodies are normal, and ask to have their levels scientifically confirmed by blood tests.

No doubt, as more information becomes available, this could become a very important field for testing. The present ranges may be further refined or adjusted. There might even be established additional ranges for new therapeutic uses, as they are discovered. We might also find a longer list of problem conditions associated with levels below, as well as with levels above, the normal ranges.

Today, it is not yet possible to test for the levels of all known vitamins; nor have all the normal ranges yet been established. But there are many important vitamin tests which can reveal certain clinical conditions, especially in combination with other laboratory tests as part of an overall health evaluation. The results may sometimes come as a surprise, since the amounts of vitamins we get in our diet may not always be reflected in the amounts found in our blood samples.

In persons who eat a balanced diet, most vitamin deficiencies are caused by faulty absorption, rather than dietary lack. This is especially true for older people. As an individual ages, the amount of stomach acid tends to decrease, affecting the ability to absorb the water-soluble vitamins. But an increased dosage is not always the right choice for such problems. For instance, a person with colitis may need more effective treatment to correct diarrhea, the cause of vitamin loss from the intestinal tract.

Some prescription medications can cause vitamin deficiencies. For example, women taking oral contraceptive pills may show decreased levels of vitamin C and various of the B-complex factors.

The side effects from excessive consumption of vitamins should be understood before considering self-medication with vitamins. The belief that if one vitamin pill is good for you, then two pills may be even better is not always necessarily true—and may actually be counterproductive and harmful.

---

*Vitamin A*
Normal range: 25 to 60 micrograms per 100 milliliters (mcg/100 ml)

Vitamin A is also known as retinol. In case you have heard vitamin A referred to as carotene, that is the precursor, found in many green and yellow vegetables, from which the vitamin is made by the body. Among the most concentrated sources of vitamin A are polar bear liver and the oil obtained from fish liver, such as cod liver oil.

The main problem associated with vitamin A deficiency in adults is a lack of night vision. In children, vitamin A deficiency can additionally lead to a failure of the bones to develop properly. This can even cause complications of the central nervous system, because the nerves and related tissues continue to grow after the vitamin A–deficient bones have stopped. Many of the nerves pass through tunnels in or between bones and can become pinched.

If as a child you were practically force-fed cod liver oil, now you know the reason. Many vitamin A deficiencies, however, are caused by faulty absorption from the intestines rather than from a dietary lack.

For both children and adults, a lack of vitamin A can lead to other complications. The skin and mucous membranes can become affected, with the skin becoming dry and scaly. As the mucous membranes dry out, they may become more susceptible to infections. Some people may even lose some of their sense of smell and taste.

Although the liver cells can store a certain amount of excess vitamin A, an overdose can lead to irritability, tiredness, headaches, nosebleeds, weakness, nausea, decreased thyroid gland activity, and even liver damage. Long-term effects of vitamin A overdosage can result in calcium deposits in ligaments and possible damage to cartilage and bone tissue.

Women who are taking oral contraceptive pills may often have higher than normal levels of vitamin A. However, these higher levels are not necessarily an indication of vitamin A overdose, unless they are accompanied by some of the symptoms described above.

---

*Vitamin D*
Normal: Levels of vitamin D are checked indirectly by measuring
    alkaline phosphatase, calcium, and phosphorus in the blood.

---

Most people are already familiar with vitamin D as a required fortifier of processed milk. The presence of this vitamin ensures that the calcium in the milk can be properly absorbed and incorporated into bone tissue.

Although there are other dietary sources of vitamin D, such as fish oils, egg yolks, and butter, the body can actually make some of its own supply of this vital nutrient. It is a complicated process, beginning with cholesterol, and also involving the ultraviolet wavelengths from sunlight (but not from artificial ultraviolet light). Because many people are not exposed to sufficient sunlight, the synthetic vitamin is added to the milk as an insurance of adequate vitamin D in the body.

A lack of vitamin D can be especially serious for growing children. Because of their increased need for calcium, this vitamin is necessary in larger-than-adult quantities to enable their growing bodies to utilize the calcium for normal skeletal development. Otherwise, a condition known as rickets may result, causing a softening of the bones and related deformities such as bowed legs. Muscular weakness and excessive tooth decay may be further evidence of this condition.

Too much vitamin D can also have serious consequences. The levels of calcium and phosphorus in the blood will become elevated, possibly causing nausea, loss of appetite, weight loss, constipation, and frequent urination. Kidney stones and even serious kidney damage may result from extra calcium in the urine and deposits of calcium in kidney tissues. At the same time, an excess of vitamin D may actually induce a loss of calcium from the bones in adults and children, further increasing the calcium in the blood to toxic levels.

Obviously, vitamin D is hardly something to experiment with in large doses.

## Vitamin K

Normal range: There is no direct test or range for vitamin K in the blood. The effective level of vitamin K is tested indirectly by measuring the prothrombin time, a test for the rate of blood clot formation in the test tube.

To the general public, this is one of the lesser-known vitamins. Yet it is an essential factor for making your blood clotting mechanism work properly whenever you sustain a cut or bruise.

There is usually more than enough vitamin K for your needs in a normal diet, especially in such foods as grains, leafy vegetables, and vegetable oils. Vitamin K is also produced by bacteria naturally present in the intestine.

A deficiency of vitamin K usually develops not because of a dietary lack but due to some organic disorder in the body. Bile duct obstruction, failure of the pancreas, or a number of conditions which prevent the absorption of fats from the intestine can all result in vitamin K deficiency.

The most serious consequence of such a deficiency is that it will take the blood far longer to form a clot and stop any bleeding. Even minor bumps and bruises can cause excessive loss of blood, leading to shock and possibly death.

Newborn infants sometimes suffer from a serious bleeding disease because their intestinal bacteria have not had a chance to multiply and manufacture sufficient vitamin K. By giving pregnant mothers large doses of vitamin K prior to delivery, the possibility of this disorder in the newborn can be prevented.

A similar problem can develop in persons who are on treatment with antibiotics for a long time and are being maintained on intravenous fluids. The prothrombin time reveals this condition, which is quickly reversed by an injection of vitamin K.

In circulatory disorders which require prevention of blood clot formation, the basis for treatment is the use of coumarol derivatives, which interfere with the action of vitamin K. Therapy is monitored with blood tests for prothrombin time. If the need for emergency surgery develops, vitamin K is given as an antidote and the operation can be done without fear of hemorrhage.

There are no known problems associated with consuming excessive quantities of vitamin K. However, an excess of vitamin K is not known to serve any useful purpose.

---

*Vitamin E*
Normal range: 0.5 to 2.0 milligrams per 100 milliliters (mg/100 ml)

---

This vitamin consists of a group of fat-soluble compounds known as tocopherols. These include d-alpha, d-beta, d-delta, and d-gamma tocopherols, of which d-alpha is the most active. A balanced mixture of the tocopherols is believed to be the best way to take the vitamin E group.

The need for vitamin E in human nutrition has been confirmed, although no minimum requirement has yet been established. It is believed that such foods as wheat germ, vegetable oils, and green leafy vegetables can provide whatever amounts of this vitamin we may normally need. People who have a diet high in polyunsaturated oils are believed to have higher requirements for vitamin E.

A wide variety of claims have been made for vitamin E: that it increases sexual vigor, strengthens the heart, maintains the integrity of cellular membranes, slows aging—and many others. These claims have yet to be directly documented by scientific studies in humans.

Experiments with animals do suggest that vitamin E is necessary for proper development of the fetus, and that a deficiency of vitamin E will result in a diminished vitality of sperm cells in the adult male. Long-term vitamin E deficiency in animals can cause a disorder resembling muscular dystrophy, with weakness and wasting of the limb muscles.

Very few cases of vitamin E deficiency have been documented in humans. The effects, however, appear to be similar to those in animals: muscular weakness, fragile red blood cells, and an excess of creatinine in the urine due to abnormal breakdown of muscle tissue. The lower the level of vitamin E in the bloodstream, the greater will be the destruction of red blood cells.

Vitamin E overdosage has been reported with such symptoms as tiredness, nausea, headaches, inflammatory changes in the gastrointestinal tract, and muscle weakness. Other toxic reactions include itching of the skin and a swelling of the face and breasts. The amount of vitamin E that can produce signs of overdosage varies from person to person.

## Vitamin B Complex

About a dozen different vitamins associated with the B complex have been identified to date. These are usually found together in a single food such as yeast, wheat germ, dairy products, meat, eggs, and various green and yellow vegetables. Any related factors that may remain to be discovered are most likely contained in the same foods. A balanced diet is the best assurance of getting all of the B-complex vitamins.

The B-complex vitamins are readily soluble in water. If you take large doses of B-complex supplements, you have probably noticed an increase in the yellow color which these vitamins impart to your urine. Because any excess of these vitamins will normally be excreted, few known side effects have so far been associated with any overdosage.

The deficiency of B-complex vitamins as a group has a telling effect on the nervous system. Symptoms can range from headaches, tiredness, and muscular weakness to outright psychosis. An example of this type of psychosis is that of a woman who fails to do her shopping and offers the excuse that her automobile is in the repair shop, but that the work is delayed due to an unavailable part, and so on, in a complex circular explanation, part of which is actually true. Administration of large doses of vitamin B-complex can successfully reverse this type of brain disorder.

On the other hand, going to your physician to ask for a periodic shot of vitamin B-complex because you feel tired and have a difficult time getting started in the morning is not an intelligent use of this group of vitamins. A balanced, reasonable diet is your best protection against B-complex deficiency. And, if the diet is unbalanced, even one multiple-vitamin tablet taken daily will provide all of the B complex that is normally needed.

For some of the B-complex vitamins, a recommended daily allowance has yet to be established. Side effects from a lack of choline, inositol, or para-aminobenzoic acid have been observed in animals; however, their importance in humans is only a presumption that has not been proved. A recommended daily allowance has been established for biotin and pantothenic acid, but testing to uncover troublesome deficiencies has yet to be perfected.

Deficiencies in a half-dozen other B-complex vitamins can also have serious consequences. There are standard laboratory testing procedures that are able to uncover these deficiencies. A description of each test follows:

*Vitamin B₁/Thiamine*
Normal range: 1.5 to 4.5 micrograms per 100 milliliters (mcg/100
ml)

Insufficient vitamin $B_1$, or thiamine, can lead to a serious condition
called beriberi. Beriberi is marked by general weakness, increased pulse
rate, heart palpitation, shortness of breath, a tired sensation after even
slight exertion, fluid buildup in the face and ankles, and a soreness in the
lower leg muscles. This condition is seen in countries where the main diet
is polished rice, made by a process that removes the outer coat. A switch
to unpolished rice or vitamin-fortified rice is often sufficient to prevent
the disease. Beriberi is usually not seen in our Western culture except in
chronic alcoholism. Some people are now suggesting that all alcoholic
beverages be fortified with thiamine to avoid this complication.

*Vitamin B₂/Riboflavin*
Normal range: 80 to 265 micrograms per gram of creatinine in urine
(mcg/g)

Most deficiencies of riboflavin are believed to stem from a problem
in absorption rather than a lack in the diet. This vitamin is readily found
in dairy products, meats, yeast, and nuts. The main signs of riboflavin
deficiency show up in the eyes and the skin. Bloodshot eyes, itching,
watering or burning of the eyes, and even sensitivity to light may all be
caused by a lack of $B_2$. The skin is subject to inflammation and scaling.
As a cure, very large doses of this vitamin are recommended to overcome
the absorption problem. The physician may order further tests to uncover the cause of the malabsorption if not already known.

*Vitamin B₃/Niacin*
Normal range: This vitamin is tested by measuring the metabolic
by-products of niacin in a 6-hour sample of urine. The range is
1.5 to 4.5 milligrams per gram of creatinine.

A deficiency in niacin has been primarily associated with pellagra,
although this condition may result from a deficiency of several members
of the B-complex group. Pellagra is characterized by skin irritation, a
deep red coloration of the tongue, difficulty with digestion, diarrhea, and

occasional disturbances of the nervous system. These signs are sometimes seen in people who eat corn as a major part of their diet, because corn is deficient in the amino acid tryptophane, from which the body makes niacin. Since large doses of niacin cause flushing of the skin, therapy for pellegra often includes doses of niacinamide or nicotinic acid, which are slightly different forms of the same vitamin that are better tolerated.

---

*Vitamin $B_6$/Pyridoxine*
Normal range: A 24-hour urine sample is tested for the $B_6$
    by-product, pyridoxal. A total of 35 to 55 micrograms (mcg) is
    normal.

---

Deficiencies in this vitamin are most frequently caused by certain drugs which interfere with $B_6$ activity in the body. Patients receiving isonicotinic acid hydrazide (INH) for tuberculosis may develop such pyridoxine deficiencies, and the same is true for women taking oral contraceptive pills. Some gynecologists now prescribe vitamin $B_6$ supplements along with the pill. Deficiency symptoms include skin and eye irritations and an upset intestinal tract similar to that caused by pellagra. Infants who are not fed adequate amounts of this vitamin may have convulsions. Adverse effects from the lack of $B_6$ in the diet of adults have not been reliably observed. Recently, there have been various claims that megadoses of vitamin $B_6$ can do wonders for one's emotional outlook.

---

*Folic Acid*
Normal range: 5 to 20 nanograms per milliliter (ng/ml)

---

Folic acid deficiency can lead to anemia, decreased white blood cell counts, and, in children, to poor growth. Since this vitamin is produced by intestinal bacteria and is also present in a wide variety of foods, a dietary deficiency of folic acid is not common. If an individual does have such a deficiency because of a poor diet or intestinal malfunction, a megaloblastic anemia can develop within six months. Persons with chronic colitis tend to lose folic acid in the stool and can develop this condition unless treated on a daily basis with folic acid tablets. Sulfa drugs cause the same problem by preventing the production of folic acid by bacteria in the intestines. The test for folic acid, which can be done accurately by radioassay, is often performed when an unexplained anemia has been discovered. Low folic acid levels may show up months before anemia develops.

---

*Vitamin B$_{12}$*
Normal range: 300 to 1,000 picograms per milliliter (pg/ml)

---

Until the discovery of synthetic vitamin B$_{12}$ in 1948, a deficiency of this vitamin often proved fatal in the disease known as pernicious anemia (see page 89). The administration of vitamin B$_{12}$ to such patients can bring about dramatic improvement in a relatively short time. The highest concentration of vitamin B$_{12}$ is in red meats, especially liver. People on strict vegetarian diets can develop pernicious anemia as a result of insufficient B$_{12}$ in the food they eat. The usual reason for pernicious anemia, however, is the inability of the body to absorb vitamin B$_{12}$ from the intestinal tract due to a lack of Intrinsic Factor, a substance that is made by the stomach lining and is responsible for transporting vitamin B$_{12}$ from the intestines into the bloodstream. Large doses of vitamin B$_{12}$ taken orally would generally prove ineffective against pernicious anemia because they would never make it into the bloodstream. That is why the vitamin is best administered by intramuscular injection, thus bypassing the need for Intrinsic Factor.

---

*Vitamin C*
Normal range: 0.2 to 2.0 milligrams per 100 milliliters (mg/100 ml)

---

Probably more has been written about vitamin C—known as ascorbic acid—than any other vitamin. There are all sorts of claims concerning its therapeutic effects in large doses. Vitamin C can supposedly prevent or reduce the effects of colds and viral influenza; it is proposed as the drug of choice in many urinary infections and to help prevent bladder cancer; it is reputed to have a beneficial effect on other forms of cancer, as well as on many serious degenerative conditions. Much of the supporting data, at this stage, is subjective, based more on individual opinions and beliefs than on scientific results.

What is known about vitamin C—and has been known for a long time—is that a lack of it can result in scurvy. This disease is marked by bleeding gums, loosening of the teeth, enlarged and bleeding hair follicles, pain in the joints, hemorrhaging under the skin, and anemia. But the quantities of vitamin C needed to prevent scurvy are quite small.

British sailors during the nineteenth century could stave off this disease by getting their entire supply of vitamin C from an occasional lime, stored aboard ship.

Since vitamin C is soluble in water, any excess is normally excreted in the urine with no ill effects. However, if an individual consumes large quantities of vitamin C and then decides to stop, a condition similar to scurvy—known as rebound scurvy—can develop. This is especially true for pregnant women. In some people, especially those with uric acid elevations, excessive amounts of vitamin C may lead to the formation of bladder and kidney stones. Diarrhea and skin rashes have also been reported. Vitamin C may interfere with anticoagulant therapy. There are indications that unless the vitamin C is fresh and well preserved, it can break down into compounds that have a whole range of unfavorable effects in different individuals.

# 11
# Testing Your Mineral Levels

As with vitamins, the evaluation of minerals in your body is often done as part of an overall assessment of your nutritional status. Such major mineral constituents as calcium, sodium, potassium, and iron are considered to be so important to your health that evaluations of their levels in your bloodstream are routinely performed as part of your normal tests (see Chapter 5).

Another category, trace minerals, is beginning to attract increasingly more attention. Present in minute quantities, they often play very important roles in the proper functioning of the body.

Trace minerals for which tests are commonly performed include chromium, copper, magnesium, manganese, selenium, and zinc. Other trace minerals are likely to earn attention among researchers, and urine and blood tests to measure their levels will probably be introduced.

Important as it may be to your health to have these trace minerals in adequate quantities, any excesses could prove quite toxic or even fatal. But there are other minerals for which people are often tested, whose presence in any amount is not beneficial. Because of our polluted environment, these highly poisonous minerals have been showing up with increased frequency in our bodies. Among them are arsenic, cadmium, lead, and mercury. Sometimes, especially in the case of suspected arsenic poisoning, the testing may be done for legal investigative purposes.

One other highly toxic mineral increasingly tested for is lithium. This mineral usually is not absorbed from the environment, but is administered as an effective drug against certain kinds of cyclic depression. Because of its toxicity, the levels of lithium in the blood must be continually monitored during therapy.

The study of minerals in the body can be done with blood or urine samples by means of a special analytical device called an atomic absorption spectrometer. This device is capable of measuring very minute quantities. The results for the mineral concentration in the blood and urine, however, may not be truly representative of the amounts stored in the tissues of the body. The blood and urine may at that time be relatively free of some of the toxic minerals, while in other tissues there could be hidden deposits that could prove lethal if they happened to get dislodged.

For this reason, interest has developed in analyzing body hair or even fingernail clippings to assess the storage of mineral constituents in the body. Hair is a part of the total body system and will incorporate, to some extent, the nutrients ingested over a period of time. Since hair grows slowly, it can present a picture of the past state of the body's mineral contents, much as tree rings reflect past growth events.

Although research performed with hair analysis is encouraging, many problems still exist in interpreting hair analysis results and in correlating these with actual disease processes. Establishing normal mineral values in hair is in itself difficult. There may be major differences in mineral contents of hair depending on the person's age, hair color, and sex. If your hair is tested and there are only slight abnormalities, it may be difficult to conclude with any certainty whether you really do have a health problem, either with mineral toxicity or mineral deficiency. If, however, your hair results are significantly elevated—or if there is a relative absence of essential trace minerals—this could be a reliable confirmation of health problems.

As more research is conducted in the correlation of hair and nail mineral assays with actual mineral levels in the various organs, some of the medical disorders whose origins remain unknown today may be explained with greater certainty in the future.

The values given with the following mineral tests are for blood or urine specimens, whichever is used more commonly for the test in question. For hair or nail sample results, it is best to refer to the normal ranges indicated by the testing laboratory on your report.

---

*Chromium*
Normal range: 5 to 20 micrograms per 100 milliliters (mcg/100 ml)

---

Chromium is not just something that makes your car's bumper shine. Although the full story on the role of chromium in the body is not yet in, it is known that the trace amounts in the diet are related to the proper functioning of insulin. Insulin is the hormone which enables the body to convert the sugar, bread, potatoes, and other carbohydrates that we eat into energy (see page 44). There is evidence that chromium enhances the effects of insulin on sugar utilization by the cells of the body. Some nutritionists are recommending that people with diabetes include in their diets foods that are high in chromium, such as whole grains and yeast.

Chromium in another form can be injected into a patient for use as a diagnostic tool. Because of its ability to label red blood cells, radioactive chromium can be used to detect loss of blood into the gastrointestinal tract, hemolytic syndromes, and survival rates of red blood cells.

Possible side effects from an excess of chromium remain under study.

---

## Copper
Normal range: 80 to 175 micrograms per 100 milliliters (mcg/100 ml)

---

Copper is a trace mineral required by certain enzymes in the body to make some of the key chemical processes work. In the thyroid gland, for example, copper is required by the enzyme for converting iodide, which the gland cannot use, into iodine, which it can use.

Some people who suffer from arthritis wear copper bracelets and claim that they help reduce the disabilities associated with their disease. There is evidence suggesting that aspirin may combine with copper in the intestinal wall and thus produce its anti-inflammatory action.

Copper deficiencies are sometimes seen in babies who are given only milk for nourishment. These infants may develop anemia because they do not have enough copper in their intestinal walls. The copper is needed to assist in the absorption of iron from the food they eat. The anemia is a result of the decreased iron concentration in the blood, which, in turn, was caused by the low levels of copper.

Copper is normally found in sufficient quantities in the foods you eat, especially in oysters, liver, whole grains, and legumes such as beans and peas. Low blood copper may not be due simply to poor nutrition but may be caused by inadequate absorption from the intestinal tract. Copper deficiency may cause bone alterations similar to those seen in scurvy, along with anemia and a decreased white blood cell count.

Increased levels of copper may develop in the blood during pregnancy, infections, heart attacks, rheumatoid arthritis, hyperthyroidism, cirrhosis, and certain types of malignancies.

In the bloodstream, copper is carried by a protein called ceruloplasmin. Many of the conditions which result in increased levels of copper are also accompanied by increased levels of ceruloplasmin.

Among the conditions associated with decreased levels of ceruloplasmin is a rare condition called Wilson's disease. Genetically related, Wilson's disease is marked by increased deposits of copper in many tissues of the body. This happens because there is not enough ceruloplasmin to keep the copper in the bloodstream. Blood levels of copper will appear below normal, since the mineral is being shunted off to the liver, kidneys, brain, and eyes. The edge of the cornea of the eye may accumulate enough copper to cause a brown ring to become visible. When a physician recognizes this sign, the Kayser-Fleischer ring, a ceruloplasmin test is indicated to confirm the diagnosis.

In advanced stages of Wilson's disease, which usually appear after the age of forty, cirrhosis of the liver may develop with serious complications. There may also be neurological problems such as loss of coordination and tremors. But if the problem is diagnosed early enough, the life of the patient can be improved and extended by the use of drugs which are capable of binding copper ions and removing them from the affected parts of the body.

---

*Magnesium*
Normal range: 1.6 to 2.6 milliEquivalents per liter (mEq/L)

---

Magnesium is another trace mineral needed by the body's enzymes to do their job. A very small amount of magnesium can go a long way in activating the large number of enzymes involved in protein and carbohydrate metabolism.

Exactly how much magnesium the body does need has yet to be established. If you eat a balanced diet, including vegetables and meat, you are most likely getting enough of this mineral. Peanuts are exceptionally high in magnesium. Any excess magnesium that your body does not need will normally be excreted in your urine and feces.

Magnesium deficiencies can develop as a result of improper diet, chronic treatment with intravenous fluids, or loss of the mineral due to excessive diarrhea or vomiting without adequate replacement. Neuromuscular difficulties, such as twitching or quivering, are usually the first signs of magnesium deficiency. If the blood level falls to 1 milliequivalent per liter or less, these problems can become more serious. Tetany-like irritability caused by noise or visual stimulation and even semi-coma leading to death can result if the condition is left untreated. Administration of adequate magnesium helps overcome these difficulties, provided it is given by injection, since magnesium salts taken by mouth are generally insoluble and cannot be used by the body.

If a patient is on intensive diuretic therapy requiring additional potassium, the physician will also be on the alert for magnesium deficiency. If that occurs, potassium therapy alone will prove ineffective, thereby seriously complicating the patient's condition unless magnesium is replaced.

Maintaining a proper balance between magnesium and calcium is very important for your body. A lack of magnesium can cause problems similar to those caused by low calcium. This is because magnesium activates the enzymes that produce parathyroid hormone, which is needed to regulate blood calcium levels. With low blood magnesium, there is a possibility of developing low blood calcium because of insufficient parathyroid hormone.

Too much magnesium is also not good for you. An excess amount acts as a sedative and can even cause the heart to stop beating. This toxicity of magnesium can be counteracted by administering calcium to revive the patient. Most of the magnesium mineral supplements now on the market come in combination with calcium. Of course, in taking them, you might also want to ask yourself what that might do to your level of phosphorus, which must also remain in a delicate balance with calcium.

---

*Manganese*
Normal range: 15 to 50 micrograms per 100 milliliters (mcg/100 ml)

---

Manganese should not be confused with magnesium. The enzymes stimulated by manganese are different from those stimulated by magnesium. Manganese is essential for the synthesis of thyroid hormone, for the function of certain peptidases that break down proteins, and for other essential metabolic reactions.

The daily requirement of manganese has not yet been precisely established. Since manganese is contained in practically every food, most people do not develop a deficiency because of a dietary lack. The absorption of manganese from the intestine is very limited even under normal conditions, and this may be the key to any deficiencies.

A deficiency in manganese can affect sugar metabolism, mimicking a diabetic condition. In certain animals, a lack of manganese can cause sterility in the males and abnormal fetal development during pregnancy, with eventual absorption of the fetus within the uterus. Similar effects have not been demonstrated in humans.

Low manganese levels are generally seen in people with epilepsy, and often in their relatives as well. Whether the manganese deficiency causes seizures, or is caused by them, has not been resolved.

Excess manganese can lead to tremors similar to those of Parkinson's disease, and to increased nervousness, anxiety, or other nervous system symptoms that are curiously similar to those caused by low magnesium. High levels of manganese also appear to inhibit the absorption of iron. If this condition persists over a prolonged period of time, anemia can result. Such disorders have been mainly limited to workers in manganese mines and can be avoided by protective measures.

---

*Selenium*
Normal range: Less than 100 micrograms per liter of urine (mcg/l)

---

Selenium is a trace mineral primarily found in shellfish, meats, egg yolks, leafy green vegetables, and grain foods.

Although not much is known about the beneficial effects of selenium in humans, trace amounts may be required by certain enzymes found in the heart and other muscles. Along with vitamin E, selenium acts to protect the liver against destruction of its cells caused by exposure to diets rich in unsaturated fats.

Selenium is readily absorbed in the intestine and transported to all parts of the body. It can be found in such tissues as liver, kidney, nails, and hair.

Inadequate amounts of selenium are thought to be associated with the early onset of aging and certain degenerative diseases. In mice and chickens, a lack of the mineral results in a condition similar to muscular dystrophy. As more research into the effects of trace minerals is performed, undoubtedly the importance of selenium to the human body will be elucidated.

An excess of selenium can be toxic to the body. Such conditions as liver disorders, fatigue, irritability, and even loss of hair could be partly due to excessive consumption of selenium.

---

*Zinc*
Normal range: 90 to 170 micrograms per 100 milliliters (mcg/100 ml)

---

As with other trace minerals, zinc is essential for activating still another array of enzymes involved in the metabolism of proteins, of nucleic acids, and of other vital processes in your body.

Zinc is involved in the production and storage of insulin in the pancreas, and in maintaining healthy skin tissue. Zinc deficiency could contribute to the onset of diabetes in adults and delayed healing of skin after it is damaged. Zinc is even used as part of the therapy for patients suffering extensive burns.

Examples of isolated zinc deficiencies, marked by an inability to satisfactorily taste food, have been described in the United States. Such deficiencies have frequently been corrected with oral zinc supplements. In severe zinc deficiencies, there may be retarded growth in both sexes and a failure of pubertal development in the male. These kinds of zinc deficiencies have been most frequently observed in the Middle East.

One reason for the arrested pubertal development is that zinc is involved in the production of the male hormone, testosterone. In fact, the testes and surrounding tissues have the highest concentration of zinc in the entire body. Whether or not zinc can also act as an aphrodisiac has not been shown; however, it so happens that one of the traditional aphrodisiac foods, namely oysters, also contains the highest concentration of zinc.

Zinc is also believed to be essential to the proper functioning of the prostate gland. In some patients with chronic prostatitis, low zinc concentrations have been found in the hair. Therapy with zinc compounds may sometimes help such patients, provided there is no other disorder involved.

Some people have a genetic disorder known as hyperzincemia. They may suffer from drowsiness and similar symptoms. The condition may also be found in industrial situations where people work with zinc. However, most people are not likely to develop hyperzincemia from overdosing with zinc supplements.

## Cadmium
Normal range: 2 to 20 micrograms per liter of urine (mcg/l)

Cadmium is toxic to the body, with no beneficial effects from even the minutest quantities. Air pollution has sharply increased the presence of cadmium in our environment. The smoking of cigarettes can further add to the level of cadmium in your body.

Even at low concentrations, cadmium is a very potent stimulator of high blood pressure. In experimental animals, cadmium is capable of doubling the systolic blood pressure in a short period of time.

Cadmium can also interfere with the activity of zinc in the body. If the ratio of cadmium to zinc is high, the patient may develop many of the problems associated with low zinc, including chronic prostatitis. Moreover, animal studies show that high cadmium-to-zinc ratios can result in damage to the sperm-producing tubules in the testicles. Whether the metal plays a similar role in human infertility remains to be determined.

The test for cadmium is not done frequently at present. As more information becomes available on the importance of zinc and the potential harm from cadmium, this test may become increasingly useful in explaining some seemingly mysterious clinical conditions.

## Lead
Normal range: Blood levels of 0 to 20 micrograms per 100 milliliters (mcg/100 ml) can be considered normal. Higher levels, beyond 20 to 40 micrograms, are considered to be a sign of overexposure to lead. In children, levels in excess of 70 micrograms per 100 milliliters require emergency treatment if complications are to be avoided.

Lead is a heavy metal which is toxic to the body. Most people are familiar with the dangers of lead poisoning. There are periodic stories of emergency treatment for children who have eaten lead-based paint or of a family getting sick from cooking with a lead-lined pot that has not been properly glazed. And we are all aware of the impact of the government's efforts to switch us from leaded to unleaded fuels.

No matter how careful you may be, you probably will have at least some lead in your blood. That is because there is lead in our environment. We either breathe it in or take it in from the foods we eat, which in turn pick it up from the soil, from the air, and, in the case of animals, from the feed they consume.

Lead poisoning can occur rapidly from consuming large portions of lead-based materials. Or it can develop slowly. Because the body will accumulate the lead that is ingested, lead poisoning can develop from small portions taken in over a long period of time.

Lead is carried by the blood to many different organs and also deposited in the bones. A high level of calcium in the blood promotes the storage of lead in the bones, which is less harmful than dispersed deposits elsewhere in the body. Low calcium or more acidic blood will favor the release of the metal from the bones. The lead will then become available to damage tissue cells by combining with cellular enzymes and causing interference with their activity.

Some of the first physical symptoms of lead poisoning are a metallic taste in the mouth, a burning sensation in the throat, vomiting, and intestinal cramps. With chronic poisoning, there is weight loss, anemia, back pain, headaches, weakness, constipation, and various neurological signs.

Because lead damages the production of hemoglobin in the bone marrow, one of the first biochemical signs of lead toxicity is a porphyria condition which turns the urine reddish brown. This is caused by some of the chemicals involved in hemoglobin synthesis appearing in the urine as abnormal by-products. When tested, the urine will show high levels of porphyrins.

The government has spent a great deal of money in sponsoring lead screening programs, especially among children, who tend to eat loose flakes of old paint often found in substandard housing. There is mounting evidence that even slightly increased levels of lead in children can cause reduced performance on intelligence tests. If detected early, medications can be used to bind the lead and extract it from the body.

---

*Arsenic*
Normal range: Any amount above 100 micrograms in a 24-hour
  urine collection is considered a sign of arsenic poisoning.

---

Arsenic is another heavy metal which is highly toxic to your body. Over the years, arsenic has figured prominently in movies and on stage as the poison of choice used by villains.

Arsenic is used as a regular component of many common pesticides and insecticides. Most of the fruits and vegetables that we eat have been sprayed with an arsenical. If only for that reason, they should be carefully washed.

Arsenic contamination can take place through the skin, by inhaling droplets sprayed in the air, and by eating materials containing arsenic.

The symptoms of acute arsenic poisoning include nausea, vomiting, diarrhea, and possible circulatory failure. When contamination takes place gradually over a long period of time, the toxic side effects are lesions on the skin, white lines appearing in the fingernails, intestinal and stomach problems, fatigue, muscle weakness, and even personality changes and mental incapacity.

It is believed that Napoleon was slowly killed by unknowingly ingesting arsenic over a prolonged period of time. Through hair analysis, a level in excess of ten times the so-called normal was found in Napoleon's hair. No one knows "who dunit."

Hair begins to concentrate arsenic within the first twenty-four to thirty hours after exposure. Fingernails and toenails also take up and store arsenic. Although nail and hair testing is becoming more common for arsenic, urine testing is what is still most commonly done. Testing the stomach juices in cases of suspected acute arsenic poisoning is also a highly useful and rapid technique.

---

## Mercury

Normal range: Levels in excess of 50 micrograms in a 24-hour urine collection indicate mercury contamination.

---

Most people are familiar with mercury as the shiny metal in thermometers and barometers. Or they may have periodically read reports of mercury contamination of tuna and other fish.

Mercury is a heavy metal increasingly found in our environment as a waste product from industrial processes. A form of mercury is also used in some medications, although far less now than it was thirty or more years ago, when it was considered to be one of the most effective components of many skin ointments.

People may become contaminated with mercury by eating it, through skin contact, and especially through breathing it. On exposure to air, the shiny liquid metal of pure mercury forms invisible fumes. This can easily happen when a thermometer or barometer breaks and the mercury disperses into elusive, tiny droplets that find their way into cracks in the flooring or into sink drains. Any such spill of mercury could present a hazard as the fumes are released. Careful decontamination is important. Mercury must never be used as a plaything despite its interesting properties.

How about the mercury contained in the "silver" fillings in your teeth? You do not need to worry. This form of mercury compound is stable and cannot generate mercury vapor. The only risk is to your dentist, who has been warned to cover the mercury supply and handle it with care.

Mercury contamination is most commonly diagnosed through urine samples. Blood samples may fluctuate too much and are not consistent enough with toxicity symptoms. In fact, even with urine tests, onset of toxic signs may vary dramatically from person to person. Some people with urine mercury levels of 500 micrograms per twenty-four hours may not show any signs of poisoning; others with levels of 100 to 200 micrograms may already have severe symptoms.

The symptoms of acute mercury toxicity are a burning taste, stomach pains, vomiting, restlessness, mental confusion, and even coma. With long-term poisoning, the signs are tremors, unsteady gait, and other neurological disorders.

It takes the body at least two months to eliminate even half of the mercury in the body. Detoxification thus is a lengthy process, with substantial amounts remaining in the body long after the source of contamination has been eliminated.

---

## Lithium

Normal range: For individuals on lithium therapy, blood levels
should be kept between 0.6 and 1.0 milliEquivalents per liter.

---

Lithium salts are not normally present in the body in significant amounts. This test is performed only for people undergoing treatment with lithium.

During the past decade lithium has been gaining increased acceptance for helping control manic-depressive mental disorders. Since it can be highly toxic to the human body, lithium must be administered in carefully controlled doses. Frequent lithium tests are performed to guard against overdosage as well as to ensure that blood levels are sufficient for therapeutic benefits.

When the lithium level rises above 1.5 milliEquivalents per liter, the first mild signs of toxicity usually become evident. These may include mental confusion and an unsteady gait. With levels above 2 milliEquivalents, the symptoms become more severe. There may be nausea, vomiting, diarrhea, thirst, frequent urination, muscle weakness and twitching, possible convulsions, and even death if lithium medication is not stopped in time. Should blood levels exceed 5 milliEquivalents per liter, fatal toxicity may occur rather quickly.

Lithium tends to replace sodium and potassium in the body. People who are on lithium therapy lose sodium and potassium in the urine. The loss of potassium is what causes frequent urination as well as an abnormal heartbeat.

When lithium medication is stopped, the body will eliminate the lithium very quickly. Within twenty-four hours, half of the lithium will be removed. On starting medication, it usually takes about a week to reach the desired therapeutic level of approximately 0.8 milliEquivalents per liter in the blood.

# 12
# Testing Your Heart Attack Risk

You may have already read the sections on blood pressure, cholesterol, and triglycerides, with their emphasis on related cardiovascular problems. So why do you need another, even more detailed chapter on this subject?

The reason is that heart disease is *the* leading cause of death in the United States today. Some 700,000 people die from heart attacks each year, often without prior warning.

The heart is an incredibly hard-working muscle. Each day it contracts about 100,000 times with a continuous rhythm to pump the blood necessary for nourishing every cell in your body. Whether you are awake or asleep, the only chance your heart gets to rest is during the less than one second between beats.

Much time, money, and effort in the past few years have been devoted to studying the factors that affect the risks of developing some form of heart disease. The federal government has sponsored a major, ongoing investigation known as the Framingham Heart Study. This project has undertaken to closely monitor a large number of inhabitants in the town of Framingham, Massachusetts, for the purpose of statistically relating the incidences of heart disease in the population to various suspected causes.

The risk factors so far identified by the Framingham Study as important contributors to heart disease are high blood pressure, cigarette smoking, and an elevated level of cholesterol. It is this study which has identified HDL cholesterol as the desirable kind and the LDL cholesterol as the one closely related to heart attacks, when present in high proportion to HDL cholesterol. These findings have been confirmed elsewhere.

Other investigators are finding that the factors identified in the Framingham Study may not be the only important ones. Some of these investigators believe that the overall behavior pattern, which they categorize as Type A or Type B, is the most important factor in determining whether an individual is likely to suffer a heart attack.

The high-risk behavior group is termed Type A and the low-risk group, Type B. The Type B individual is generally more relaxed and "laid back" than the Type A, who is more intense, driving, and aggressive. Type A individuals are much more likely to become angry about details that elude their control. Just driving home from work in slow traffic or waiting in a long line at the grocery checkout counter can easily raise their level of frustration.

Most individuals who suffer from heart attacks fall into the Type A category. The risk factors of smoking, elevated cholesterol, and high blood pressure may even be absent in such people, although these factors often compound their problem.

Whether we happen to fit the Type A or Type B pattern is influenced partly by the times we live in, by our set of values, and by our inheritance —both psychological and genetic—from our parents. Moreover, if both our parents lived a long life, the chances favor that we may have the same experience. If both our parents died of degenerative diseases at an early age, we may be up against tougher odds to reach a ripe old age.

But keep in mind that in evaluating heart disease risks, these and other factors are interpreted in the context of statistical probabilities— or the odds of coming down with a problem under certain conditions. We are not dealing with the certainty of a particular event. No one has yet been able to assure anyone with absolute certainty of a long life— or condemn anyone to an early death—on the basis of statistics.

Many people are eager to do their utmost to improve their chances for a healthy life and reduce their risk of heart attack. There is nothing they can do about their genetic inheritance, and there may be little they can do to change themselves from a Type A personality to a Type B. But they can do a lot to improve or eliminate some of the other factors identified by the Framingham Study as increasing their chances of a heart attack. They can give up smoking; they can lower their cholesterol by exercising, changing their diets, and otherwise improving their lifestyles.

Millions of people are already doing so, with dramatically positive results. Heart attack rates in the United States appear to be on the way down. The desire for physical self-improvement may turn out to be one of the most significant revolutions in our nation's history, with far-ranging effects on our lives and our institutions.

Yet for some people, such efforts may turn out to be counterproductive. The psychological and physical stress of actually changing their lifestyle may impose an unacceptable burden on their system. It is possible that for these relatively few individuals, the means may not justify the desired end of reducing the likelihood of heart disease. That is why informed prudence may be the best policy before doing something drastic in this area.

What are *your* odds of coming down with a heart attack? Obviously, you and your physician are in the best position to evaluate your genetic inheritance and your psychological disposition. But there are tests which can definitely give you some measurable indications, some objective yardstick by which you can gauge your own cardiovascular health.

To begin with, you may want to review the sections on high blood pressure (page 26), cholesterol (page 55), and triglycerides (page 58). These can serve as an introduction to other aspects of those tests that will be discussed in this chapter, as well as to the laboratory procedure known as lipoprotein phenotyping.

Also included in this chapter is a section on electrocardiogram stress testing, even though it is not strictly a laboratory procedure. Stress testing is being increasingly done as a way of further assessing cardiovascular health.

## "Good" and "Bad" Cholesterol

That cholesterol can play an important role in heart attacks has been established by the Framingham Study. The exact process of how this happens is not yet known, but some facts have become apparent.

It is believed that plaques containing about 40 to 50 percent of fatty substances, made up mainly of cholesterol, are deposited within the walls of the blood vessels. As more fatty materials are deposited, the plaques become larger and intrude into the channel of the blood vessel.

What follows is somewhat like a chain reaction. Platelets, which help to make your blood clot, circulate in the bloodstream and strike those obstructions. The platelets react by sticking to the plaques. In turn, these surface accumulations of platelets can trap more cholesterol—as well as triglycerides—until the flow of blood becomes restricted.

As the arteries clog up, the blood pressure rises, putting a strain on the heart muscle. If the clogging occurs in the coronary arteries of the heart, the blood supply to the heart tissue is reduced, thus depriving the heart of oxygen. If the oxygen level gets too low, the heart will form what is known as an infarct—and that portion of it will die. When this process of infarction happens quickly, the person will have the symptoms of a heart attack with severe pain, sweating, and collapse.

The result is that the damaged tissue interferes with the normal pulsation of the heart. The heart develops an irregular beating pattern called arrhythmia. If not treated promptly, this rhythm disturbance can cause sudden death—a tragic culmination to the process indirectly started by the buildup of cholesterol and other fatty substances along the lining of the blood vessels.

The normal amount of total cholesterol varies from 140 to 280 milligrams per 100 milliliters of blood serum, in most laboratories. If you have a low-normal cholesterol below 150 milligrams, there seems to be a very small chance that you will develop cardiovascular disease. If your total cholesterol is in excess of 300 milligrams, you are three to five times more likely to develop cardiovascular disease than the general population.

But that is only part of the story. The fact is that the majority of heart attacks—about 75 percent—involve individuals with a normal total cholesterol. Obviously, there must be other powerful factors at work in building toward a heart attack.

Part of the answer was supplied by the Framingham Study in its emphasis on high-density lipoproteins (HDL) and low-density lipoproteins (LDL). These are two of the three distinct and separate fractions which make up total cholesterol. VLDL, very-low-density lipoproteins, comprise the remainder. In the past several years, special techniques have been developed to measure LDL and HDL in the serum. These measurements are usually performed for any patients suspected, for various reasons, of having higher than normal risks of heart attack.

What the Framingham Study showed is that people with relatively high HDL levels had a significantly lower incidence of heart disease and strokes than the general population, whereas those with high LDL levels had a significantly higher incidence.

Why this should be so remains under investigation. However, it does appear that most of the cholesterol is transported in the LDL blood fraction. When total cholesterol is elevated, it is usually found to be the LDL type. And it is the LDL cholesterol which is found in the plaques lining the blood vessel walls.

In the general population, an HDL cholesterol value between 45 and 55 milligrams per 100 milliliters of blood is associated with an average risk of developing cardiovascular diseases. If, however, the HDL concentration is 25 milligrams or less, the risk is over twice that of the general population. On the opposite end of the scale, if the HDL level is over 70 milligrams per 100 milliliters of blood, then the risk is only one-half that of the general population.

The amount of HDL cholesterol found in women is slightly higher than that in men. And women, in general, have a lower risk of cardiovascular disease than men. Clearly, all signs indicate that the more HDL you have, the better your chances of avoiding heart trouble.

LDL cholesterol is also an important factor in assessing your cardiovascular risks. Whenever total cholesterol rises, the LDL fraction tends to rise disproportionately. The key indicator with LDL is its proportion to HDL.

The normal proportion of LDL to HDL is between 3.0 and 3.5. If that ratio reaches 6.0 in men or 5.0 in women—either because of increased LDL, decreased HDL, or a combination of both—then the chances of cardiovascular disease rise to twice that of the general population. Values over 6.0 indicate even greater risks.

According to this formula, even if your total cholesterol is on the low side, you could still be in the high-cardiovascular-risk category. For example, you could have a total cholesterol of 180 milligrams, yet if your HDL was only 25, your LDL-to-HDL ratio would be 6.0, placing you in the double-the-normal-risk category. On the other hand, you could have an elevated total cholesterol of 280, yet if your HDL was 60, you would have about a 3.4 ratio of LDL to HDL—putting you in the normal category.

The lower your LDL-to-HDL ratio, the better off you are. For people whose ratio is as low as 1.0 if they are men and 1.5 if women, the risk of cardiovascular disease drops to one-half that of the general population.

Fortunately, there are ways of reducing your LDL-to-HDL ratio by increasing your level of HDL cholesterol and at the same time reducing your LDL cholesterol. How? By jogging and other forms of exercise. An occasional alcoholic drink is reputed to have a similar effect. Such factors as salt intake, diet, age, family history, triglyceride level, smoking, and body weight may also one day be related to changes in your LDL-to-HDL ratio.

## Lipoprotein Phenotyping

The Framingham Study has so far not attempted to draw any direct link between the level of triglycerides and the incidence of heart disease. However, triglycerides were an important consideration in evaluating cardiovascular risks prior to the publication of the relatively new data on LDL and HDL cholesterol.

Studies conducted by Drs. Donald Fredrickson and Robert Levy at the National Institutes of Health in Bethesda, Maryland, in the late 1960s implicated elevated triglyceride levels with the likelihood of heart-related problems. These studies defined five basic types of disorders involving the fatty materials transported in the blood.

The test for identifying these disorders is known as lipoprotein phenotyping. Through electrophoresis fractionation this test subdivides the fatty protein substances in your blood into their components. In addition to the HDL and LDL fractions, there is a fraction labeled very-low-density lipoproteins, or VLDL, and another termed chylomicrons. Both VLDL and chylomicrons may contain varying amounts of triglycerides.

Lipoprotein phenotyping is done quite commonly and is widely considered to provide useful information on the possibility of heart disease and related circulatory disorders.

About 90 percent of the blood fat disorders uncovered by lipoprotein phenotyping fall into two of the five possible categories of disorders. These are known as Type 2 and Type 4.

The Type 2 individual has no chylomicron droplets filled with triglycerides, but can have slightly elevated triglycerides in the VLDL fraction. The total cholesterol is definitely elevated. The incidence of Type 2 people coming down with heart disease is quite high, two to three times that of the general population. The Type 2 individual is usually affected with premature severe artherosclerosis, which could lead to an early death. However, certain other conditions, such as liver and kidney diseases, hypothyroidism, porphyria, and increased globulin protein, can give the appearance of a Type 2 phenotype. The possibility of such conditions has to be eliminated prior to diagnosing anyone as having a Type 2 pattern.

The Type 4 individual has a VLDL fraction containing triglycerides that are significantly elevated, and the chylomicron triglycerides are usually slight or absent. Total cholesterol is most often normal or only slightly elevated. The incidence of cardiovascular disease for the Type 4 individual is approximately as high as for the Type 2. This is a good example of a major disorder in which the level of total cholesterol seems to play only a minor role.

As with Type 2, other factors can cause a Type 4 pattern. These include alcoholism, sugar diabetes, an underactive thyroid gland, gout, kidney disease, an inflamed pancreas, the taking of oral contraceptive pills, and even pregnancy.

Although both Type 2 and Type 4 carry similar risks, Type 2 is primarily due to genetic factors, while Type 4 is partly related to a particular lifestyle. The onset of Type 4 patterns usually occurs in middle age, when the intake of food exceeds the caloric requirements of a more sedentary life. The liver converts the excess calories to triglycerides, which in turn raise the VLDL fraction.

Individuals with patterns labeled Type 1, 3, or 5 all show different forms of triglyceride elevations in combination with various levels of cholesterol fractions. All three types carry significantly increased risks of cardiovascular problems, but may also be caused by other conditions. If you are among the relatively small proportion of people with these types of blood fat disorders, you should ask your physician to explain your type to you in detail.

Phenotype-pattern disorders are, for the most part, manageable through changes in diet, exercise, and treatment with various medications. The medication, diet, and other lifestyle changes should be tailored to the particular disorder identified by your pattern. By using the knowledge based on your personal phenotype pattern, your potential for coming down with cardiovascular problems because of blood fat disorders can be significantly reduced.

## Stress Testing

The traditional way of checking the health of your heart has been the electrocardiogram, or EKG. The EKG often is a part of a complete physical examination. It consists of attaching sensing electrodes to various parts of the body in order to measure the heart's electrical impulses. The impulses are recorded automatically on a graph and are then studied by the physician for any abnormalities. The test has traditionally been administered with the patient resting comfortably on an examining table in the physician's office.

Yet heart attacks do not usually occur while the victim is at rest.

On the contrary. They often take place while the victim is under stress; sometimes, extreme stress. Perhaps there was an argument, or the person was running to catch a bus, or had too much food or alcoholic beverages. We have all heard of people who had been given a clean bill of health, including an EKG, only to drop dead the next day of a heart attack.

What the stress test seeks to do is to measure the functioning of the cardiovascular system while re-creating the conditions of physical stress under controlled circumstances. The idea is that any abnormalities are much more likely to show up during a stress test than under the relaxed conditions of a normal EKG.

Increasingly, more health-conscious people are requesting the stress test—and incurring a considerable expense—as a check on their physical conditioning program. A physician may recommend a stress test as a safety precaution to individuals planning to undertake some new form of strenuous exercise. And sedentary individuals with normal EKGs—and no intention of taking up exercise—may sometimes be put through a stress test if their physician suspects that they might have a hidden cardiovascular problem because of their laboratory tests or symptoms of chest pain.

The stress test involves monitoring a person's EKG, pulse rate, and blood pressure first at rest, and then while on a treadmill. If any abnormalities show up while at rest, the treadmill exercise may not be desirable because of the risk of injury to the heart.

If, however, everything appears normal, the person is asked to walk on the treadmill belt. The belt initially moves at a natural walking pace, almost horizontal to the floor. Gradually, the belt's speed is increased and the angle is made steeper.

The individual continues this form of exercise up to the point of exhaustion. The total time on the treadmill may be fifteen to twenty minutes. With some people who are in good condition, the angle of the belt and its speed may approximate running uphill at a fast jog.

While on the treadmill, the person is continuously monitored by EKG and measured for pulse rate and blood pressure in the presence of a physician. Should any abnormality develop—such as an irregular EKG pattern or chest pains—the exercise would be stopped immediately.

The data of the stress test are reviewed for the purpose of counseling the individual on the degree of physical exertion that may be safely tolerated. If the results are abnormal, the physician will have to investigate not only the immediate cause of the problem, but also the underlying factors, which may include remote or subtle disease conditions. The results may also indicate what treatment—such as weight reduction or gradual exercise conditioning or special medication—may be most appropriate.

The stress test may not uncover all possible cardiovascular irregularities. But along with your other laboratory tests and physical examination results, it serves to further round out the picture of how well your heart is likely to serve you in the years to come.

# 13
# Testing for Common Infections

It could be something as common as a sore throat, diarrhea, or athlete's foot. Or it could be something far more serious, such as tetanus or blood poisoning. What all these conditions have in common is that they are caused by microscopic organisms.

Microscopic organisms are virtually everywhere; not only in the spray from the person sneezing uncomfortably close to you, but also in the water you drink, the food you eat, the air you breathe, the things you touch. They are present in many parts of your body, from your skin to some of your innermost body cavities.

Fortunately, not all microscopic organisms cause disease. Most are quite harmless. Many others are even beneficial in certain parts of the body—but harmful if found elsewhere. A peaceful organism from the rectum may wreak havoc in the urinary tract. Still other microorganisms are harmful no matter where they are.

Infections by these harmful "bugs" are the ones we are concerned about. There are literally hundreds of different disease-causing agents, and they usually fall into one of the general categories known as bacteria, viruses, fungi, and parasites.

A phase of laboratory testing known as microbiology seeks to specifically identify the offending microorganisms in a given disease condition. The purpose of such testing is to confirm the physician's diagnosis and treatment—or to change it. In some infections, treatment cannot even begin until the identity of the offending agent is known.

With many of the more common infections, such as a sore throat or diarrhea, your doctor's diagnosis will hardly come as a surprise. But there are many other infections which may not be so obvious. You may merely have a fever, feel a general malaise, or experience weight loss. It may take a complete physical examination, with a full battery of screening tests, before your physician can diagnose your problem as an infection.

What kind of infection? Again, with most cases of visible infection, your doctor will have a pretty good idea as to what it may be on the basis of his or her diagnostic experience. If the infection is diagnosed partly on the basis of a complete blood count, the white blood cells will be elevated if the infection is bacterial. A high eosinophil level may indicate intestinal parasites. A normal or low total white cell count with an increased lymphocyte level could suggest that the infection is caused by a virus.

To identify which organism is responsible for the problem, a sample is taken from the affected area and sent to the laboratory for analysis. This sample may be made by touching a cotton swab to the back of the throat, or collecting a scraping of scales from the skin, a drop of pus from a skin infection, an ounce of "clean catch" urine, a fresh stool specimen, or a blood sample taken after careful disinfection of the skin over a vein.

## How the Tests Are Done

On the basis of your doctor's preliminary diagnosis and the kind of sample sent for study, the laboratory knows whether to test the sample for bacteria, viruses, fungi, or parasites. This information is very important because the tests for each of these general categories are quite different.

Bacteria are by far the most frequent subjects of microbiological testing in laboratories. There are two steps in bacterial identification. First, the bacteria are cultured, which means that they are grown in quantity in order to obtain enough organisms to find out whether they are a harmful kind—or whether they merely represent the normal inhabitants or flora of the region of the body from which the specimen was taken.

If it is determined that they are indeed a harmful type, one or more of the colonies of bacteria are cultured a second time. The culture media and techniques in this step are chosen to allow the specific identification of the bacteria causing the infection.

At the same time, other cultures are made in the presence of several coded paper discs saturated with various antibiotics that may be able to stop the infection. The successful antibiotics are reported to the doctor to provide a choice of treatment likely to give the best results.

The isolated bacteria may be exposed to as many as twelve specific antibiotics to see which one works the best against a pure culture. Since it usually takes an extra day to complete this work, the physician may have already prescribed a broad-spectrum antibiotic. The antibiotic-sensitivity test results may indicate that such treatment should be continued or that it be changed to a different drug.

What if your physician suspects a virus? Although viral infections are probably as common as those caused by bacteria, there are no rapid laboratory tests for viruses. For one thing, viral testing is a very lengthy and involved process which, in most cases, would be prohibitively expensive, unless the disease was a very serious one. Another problem is that by the time an identification could be made, most viral infections would have run their course. Moreover, there is no arsenal of drugs which is comparably as effective against viruses as antibiotics are against bacteria. Any treatment would still be limited to bed rest, fluids, and fever-preventing medications.

As more specific anti-viral agents are developed, new and simpler ways of identifying viruses in laboratories will also be made available. At present, a negative test result for bacterial infection indirectly confirms a clinical impression of viral infection or some other illness.

Much more frequently tested than viruses are specimens from suspected fungus or yeast infections. Although it may take two to four weeks to get a final identification, the course of most of these infections tends to be slow. Fortunately, the treatments for fungus or yeast infections are very effective. General therapy can usually be started right away, based on a preliminary examination of the specimen under a microscope, which often provides a tentative diagnosis of the major type of organism.

As for intestinal parasites, these are usually identified from stool specimens. No one likes to think of having parasites, even if such organisms do not usually approach in size the kind we can see with the naked eye.

Most intestinal parasites are microscopic in size. Only through a close examination of the stool specimen under a microscope can these parasitic organisms or their eggs be properly identified. Fresh stool specimens are critical in this type of diagnostic test, since the organisms tend to degenerate and become unrecognizable as the specimen becomes dried out.

Different microorganisms tend to infect different, very specific parts of the body. Literally hundreds of these "bugs" have been identified and volumes have been written about them. Here are some of the most common ones, categorized by where they are most likely to strike.

## Ear, Nose, and Throat Infections

Among the most common and uncomfortable of all infections are those which settle in the upper respiratory area. The nose, throat, and ears are interconnected. Any infection can migrate from one to the other, and often does.

The throat is usually the focus, or the starting point, for most such infections. The throat can become infected by viruses as well as by bacteria, but the viruses are not detectable through usual laboratory methods.

The throat is a good example of an area which normally harbors many harmless or beneficial bacteria. The throat as well as the nose is normally populated by nonpathogenic neisseria organisms and alpha-hemolytic streptococcus. The latter is actually believed to protect the throat from harmful organisms, and is not the cause of the dreaded "strep throat."

But change the name just a bit, to group A beta-hemolytic streptococcus, and you have serious problems: a strep throat and the threat of complications. The strep throat diagnosis through laboratory testing is an important distinction, since the side effects of this type of infection can cause severe heart and kidney damage.

Other harmful bacteria sometimes found in the throat are pneumococci, associated with pneumonia; *Neisseria meningitidis,* which can cause meningitis; *Staphylococcus aureus,* which is also found on the skin, where it can cause boils; and *Hemophilus influenzae,* which causes middle-ear infections and secondary lung infections. A different strain related to hemophilus is responsible for whooping cough.

Because of the nose, throat, and ear interconnection, the ears and sinus cavities can be infected by the same bacteria which infect the throat. In testing for any such infection in all three areas, the infecting organisms should be found in significant numbers for the tests to be meaningful, since a few of them could be a normal finding.

In testing for throat infections, one crucial distinction should never be missed. What looks like a "strep throat" caused by bacteria can sometimes be mononucleosis caused by a virus. Although there is no way to find the virus by doing a standard culture, the complete blood count can raise the suspicion and another blood test, called the heterophile test, can confirm it. What this test does is to analyze the body's defensive response to possible mononucleosis infection.

Fungus can also affect the throat and mouth in the disease known as thrush. Thrush is occasionally seen in young children. It is caused by the fungus *Candida albicans,* which is the same organism that infects the vaginal canal in a condition called moniliasis. Whether thrush or moniliasis, the condition can be caused by antibiotic treatment employed against bacterial infections. What happens is that the antibiotics kill off numerous beneficial bacteria along with the harmful ones. With insufficient numbers of the beneficial bacteria to populate the surface membranes, *Candida albicans* can overgrow and cause a secondary infection in the throat, in the vaginal canal, and even in the intestinal tract.

## Urinary Tract Infections

Urinary tract infections occur when harmful bacteria find their way into the urethra, from where they may migrate to the bladder and even to the kidneys. If the bacteria remain to multiply primarily in the urethra, they cause urethritis. If the bladder becomes involved, it is called cystitis. And with kidney involvement, it is pyelonephritis.

Males are more likely to develop urethritis—sometimes with prostate gland complications—because the male urethra is longer than the female urethra. But the longer urethra protects males from developing cystitis. Cystitis is more common in females, in whom the bacteria have a shorter route of travel to infect the bladder, and because the urethral opening is near sources of bacteria from the vagina and rectum.

Some of the infections occurring in the urinary tract are thought to be virtually spontaneous, with bacteria from the intestinal tract finding their way to the urinary opening. Among the offending bacteria in the urinary tract may be such normal inhabitants of the intestinal tract as E. coli, proteus, klebsiella, or enterobacter. Poor hygiene and various sexual practices can sometimes be contributory factors.

Sexual contact can introduce other infection-producing bacteria into the urinary tract. Probably the best known of these is the organism which causes gonorrhea.

But there can be other reasons for urinary tract infections, in part related to the patient's overall resistance. One unusual type is known as "honeymoon cystitis," a bladder infection which starts in young women

after frequent episodes of sexual intercourse. It is thought that the urethra becomes irritated and allows more bacteria to enter the bladder and
to set up an infection.

Symptoms of urinary tract infection can vary widely. Sometimes
there are no symptoms, especially in women. More often, there may be
burning or itching of the urethra, frequent urination, pain in the groin
or bladder area, an ache in one or both kidney areas, and a general feeling
of illness or lack of energy.

Along with an examination by a physician, a urine culture often
plays a key role in diagnosing a urinary tract infection. To get the best
possible urine sample, the physician may give the patient a small sterile
container with the instruction to return it with urine voided upon awak-
ening in the morning. This urine will have been in the bladder for many
hours, long enough to collect more bacteria, whereas urine collected
during the day may have been held only an hour or two and may fail
to reveal active infection in the urinary tract. But if the symptoms are
present, the doctor may find it advisable to collect some urine right away.

It is very important how the sample is collected, using so-called
sterile technique. In order to avoid contamination by bacteria present on
the outer surface of the body, the urine should be collected in midstream.
Otherwise, some of the usual organisms at the opening of the urinary
canal could overgrow in culture and mask the presence of a more harmful organism within the urinary tract. The collection cup should be
submitted to the laboratory as soon as possible so that the organisms do
not get a chance to multiply and misleadingly increase the number of
colonies in the urine culture.

The laboratory will isolate and grow the organisms which may be
causing the problem. A count of the bacteria will also be made, since the
seriousness of a urinary infection depends not only on the kind of bacteria present, but also on their concentration. Generally, if the number of
organisms is in excess of 100,000 per milliliter of urine, there is cause for
concern. However, with some organisms a count as low as 10,000 per
milliliter is a sign of disease, provided that clinical symptoms are present.

A routine urinalysis is often done on the same "clean" specimen to
determine whether the infection is located in the bladder or in the
kidneys. A significant number of casts in the urine sediment is an indication that the kidneys are inflamed by the infection and are releasing
proteins. If no casts are found and the urine sediment contains only
epithelial cells, the chances are that there is an infection in the lining of
the bladder.

Antibiotic sensitivity testing of the offending bacteria helps the doctor decide on the appropriate therapy. With proper antibiotic treatment, the symptoms of a urinary tract infection should ease within the first twenty-four hours. However, treatment must be continued for one week or longer to eliminate all infection.

If the symptoms persist, the medication may have to be changed by the physician. The laboratory reports show what alternative medications may be effective. Additional specimens may also have to be cultured to follow the response to the treatment and confirm the elimination of the bacteria from the urinary tract. Sometimes these follow-up cultures may reveal that more than one type of bacteria was present, with one type being able to persist after the other succumbs to a particular drug.

Some cases of urinary tract infection may develop into chronic problems, with the infection flaring up every few months, then temporarily subsiding upon treatment. Further testing and treatment monitoring may be indicated with this type of problem.

Of special importance is the possible development of antibiotic resistance, whereby the organism adapts to the medication and is able to grow again to produce harm. Another culture with antibiotic sensitivity tests can solve this problem.

## Skin Infections

The skin contains a number of various microorganisms which usually live in harmony with the body. While some are merely transient inhabitants of the skin, many other organisms exist there permanently, often helping to protect the skin in subtle ways.

In the category of bacteria, those that often cause problems for the skin are the staphylococcus and streptococcus groups. The disorders they may trigger range from acne to boils or impetigo. A culture may be needed if the infection is either long-term, such as acne, or highly virulent, such as impetigo. By knowing the identity of the harmful organism and whether it is resistant to any of the antibiotics, the most appropriate treatment can be selected.

Fungi in the skin are usually more of a nuisance than a threat to health. The fungi that lodge themselves in the moist crevices between the toes to cause the common "athlete's foot" are well known. Treatment is usually given without taking any tests if the case is mild. A scraping may be taken in stubborn cases to confirm the diagnosis and rule out other possibilities, such as allergies.

Another common skin fungus is *Tinea versicolor,* which is especially bothersome for people attempting to acquire an even suntan. The small spots affected by the fungus will remain scaly and untanned. Scrapings can be taken to confirm the tinea infection, but a special ultraviolet lamp available in most dermatologists' offices may do the job instantaneously.

In deeper wounds, such as punctures from sharp objects or animal bites, organisms of the clostridium group are of special concern. In the absence of oxygen, clostridium bacteria can multiply to cause gas gangrene or tetanus. Clostridium bacteria are widespread inhabitants of the soil and infect the body when introduced by foreign objects. A swab from such a wound, when cultured in a laboratory, can alert the physician to the problem before serious or even fatal complications develop.

## Intestinal Tract Infections

Although the acidic stomach contents are relatively free of microorganisms, the lower intestines contain a wide variety of them, ranging from bacteria to yeast cells and possibly parasites.

A major inhabitant of the intestines is the bacterium E. coli, which is harmless in its natural habitat and is in fact essential to proper elimination.

Laboratories are often asked to check for the presence of E. coli in food, milk, or water as a sign of fecal contamination. Such a finding means that other, more harmful germs—such as those causing dysentery —may be present. It is thought that the diarrhea, or "turista," that affects visitors to some tropical countries is caused by an infection of the intestinal tract with a modified strain of E. coli. These strains resemble the normal ones in culture, so that testing is not critical unless the diarrhea fails to subside with treatment.

Foods containing staphylococcus or salmonella bacteria can cause major intestinal problems. When allowed to multiply in unrefrigerated contaminated foods, staphylococcus releases poisons which cause extreme irritation to the intestinal tract. The laboratory identification of the offending organism is often made with a leftover portion of the suspected food.

While most cases of diarrhea run their course quickly, with no need to identify the causative organism, serious cases are often analyzed through cultures from stool samples. On the basis of the results, special therapeutic measures may have to be taken to save the patient. And various precautions may also be taken to keep the disease from spreading to other persons. This could be the case if the causative agent is from the shigella or vibrio groups, responsible for dysentery and cholera, respectively.

Viruses of unknown origins sometimes cause severe intestinal upsets. But these are usually of the "twenty-four-hour flu" category, and there is no way to identify them in time to be of any use. When epidemic outbreaks occur, virus cultures may be prepared in order to devise an immunization program.

Parasites which can infect the intestinal tract are a field of study unto themselves. The identification of possible parasitic infection requires a fecal specimen or, occasionally, a smear from the anal canal. The identification under a microscope is made by an experienced parasitologist, who looks for any evidence of the parasite's life cycle: eggs, cysts, larvae, or adult forms. Sometimes, however, the parasites may be of sufficient size to be visible in the stool as worms.

Amoebae, worms, and protozoa are the general groups of parasitic organisms which can cause distress in the intestinal tract. If left untreated, debilitating complications may sometimes follow. Through the laboratory identification of the parasite, an effective treatment can usually be prescribed.

## Blood Infections

The occasional presence of some bacteria in your bloodstream is not unusual and may not mean disease. By bringing its lymphatic tissue defense mechanism into play, your body will usually filter out these bacteria with no untoward side effects. In fact, you may not even know it is happening.

If, however, the bacteria multiply and reach significant numbers, a serious illness called septicemia, or blood poisoning, may occur. Unless antibiotics are given in large amounts, the body's defense system may be unable to cope with an overwhelming infection of this type.

As a rule of thumb, septicemia occurs when the microorganisms are multiplying as fast or faster than the rate at which the body can remove them. Signs of septicemia are general malaise, increased pulse rate, chills, fever, and prostration—possibly leading to collapse, or septic shock.

A blood infection can be dangerous for other reasons. Within the bloodstream, the invading germs are carried to other parts of the body. By infecting such vital organs as the brain, spinal cord, liver, kidneys, or the heart valves, the organisms could cause death.

Septicemia may be caused by many types of organisms: staphylococcus, streptococcus, neisseria, hemophilus, E. coli, and others. The invasion may take place through a wound, a deep skin infection, a lung infection, or other entrances which allow the microorganism to reach the bloodstream and multiply.

Laboratory microbiology is an integral resource in helping the physician decide how treatment should proceed in this serious disorder. Several blood culture specimens are taken before antibiotic therapy is begun. Even a single dose of an antibiotic could interfere with accurate identification of the germ by preventing its growth in the laboratory culture medium.

Life-saving antibiotics may have to be started immediately after the samples are taken if the patient's condition is critical. Once the microorganism is identified in a positive blood culture—which may take up to several days—the treatment may be adjusted accordingly. Periodic blood cultures can be taken to follow the progress of treatment by looking for the decreased numbers of the offending bacteria, and their eventual elimination from the blood.

Following successful treatment of the acute phase, attention has to be given to the possibility of chronic flare-ups. These could occur as a result of the continued presence of germs in such vital organs as the heart valves or deep within the kidneys. Appropriate medication is mobilized to control such crises and, eventually, to eliminate them.

## About Resistance to Antibiotics

We have all heard a great deal about this. The antibiotic which was effective yesterday is no longer effective today. The organisms have become stronger, in fact almost immune to the measures designed to eliminate them.

Here is where laboratory sensitivity tests are crucial. The microbiologist never assumes that just because a particular organism was susceptible to a certain antibiotic yesterday, that same antibiotic will be effective in eliminating it tomorrow. In fact, resistance to antibiotics is a constant hazard and obstruction to the expected results of current-day "wonder drugs."

A case in point is that of a child with an ear and throat infection caused by the bacteria *Hemophilus influenzae.* The child was given the usual antibiotic for this condition, but it soon became apparent that the patient was not improving. The infection spread, causing a severe abscess in the tonsil area and a swelling which even prevented opening the mouth. Thanks to laboratory testing of cultures from a throat swab, it was discovered that the organisms were highly sensitive to a totally different antibiotic, not usually used for this condition. With the change to that antibiotic, the treatment proved successful in short order. At about the same time, similar findings were being seen in other laboratories, and physicians throughout the country were alerted to the possibility that this condition may now require different treatment.

The challenge remains. Although new antibiotics continue to be discovered to treat the slightly altered, somewhat new infections of our day, we must be ready with the antibiotics of tomorrow to treat the infections of tomorrow. An indispensable partner in this quest will always be the laboratory, checking and testing whether we are adequately protected against these new threats to our health.

# 14
# A Look into the Future

Twenty-five years ago, perhaps even ten years ago, there would have been little demand for a book of this sort. The medical profession and other specialists in the field had their technical texts. But the general public was yet to be exposed to medical laboratory testing as a matter of routine. Some of the tests described as routine in this book were yet to be devised.

What would be some of the new materials in a similar book on laboratory testing ten or even twenty-five years from now?

With advances in this field coming so fast and often so unexpectedly, the nature of some of these future tests could be anybody's guess. But other advances can be predicted with more certainty. Many promising new tests are already on the drawing boards, or at different stages of evolution. Some are already in use, if not on a widespread basis. Together, they point in the general direction where tomorrow's testing is heading.

## Testing for Cancer

There is no single physical disorder which gets more attention—both from the general public and the medical profession—than cancer. The key to effective treatment is early detection; yet detection has always lagged behind advances in treatment.

Undoubtedly the day will come when a single blood or urine test will be devised to act as a screening test for all cancers. Several candidates for this distinction are already under study.

One such test is named serum TPA, for tissue polypeptide antigen. TPA is associated with a wide variety of malignant tumors; however, since TPA may increase temporarily with bacterial infections, a positive test must be repeated after several weeks. The TPA blood test is in the research stage.

Also in the research stage is the test for TAF, tissue angiogenesis factor. This substance is involved in the formation of new blood vessels necessary to nourish invasive cancers. Different methods of detecting and measuring TAF are currently being devised.

Perhaps the newest test in this field is that for GT-II, galactosyl transferase enzyme. Cancer cells seem to be dependent on a special form of this enzyme for their energy metabolism. As a result, the cancer begins to manufacture larger than normal amounts of G.T. type II enzyme in order to survive. The excess enzyme is released into the bloodstream, where it can be measured. This test has already proved positive for the detection of many types of intestinal tract cancers. It has passed the research stage, but is not convenient or reliable enough to be introduced as a clinical test. Three or more years may be needed to reach that stage.

There are other tests for specific cancers which are in use by major laboratories at this very moment. Without reliable specific tests as a follow-up, general tests for cancer could do more harm than good. Telling a person that he or she may have cancer without being able to pinpoint the site of the cancer, perhaps for years, could create excessive concern.

The most common specific cancer-detecting test is the Pap smear for women, which has already been discussed in detail (see page 139), as has a much newer PAP test for detecting cancer of the prostate gland in men (see page 141).

Other new, specific cancer-detecting tests include determination of AFP, alphafetoprotein. AFP is a substance which is normally present in the fetus—but not in the newborn. AFP reappears in the blood in cases of cancer of the liver and certain cancers of the testicles.

Another test is for CEA, carcino-embryonic-antigen, which is normally made in small amounts by the cells lining the intestinal tract. CEA is released in much larger amounts by malignant tumors of the intestines, pancreas, or bronchial tubes of the lungs. Although subject to some interference by irritative diseases such as colitis and even by cigarette smoking, this test has already proved useful in following up on patients after surgical removal of CEA-producing tumors. Any tumor cells left behind reveal their presence by producing larger than normal amounts of CEA. A recurrence of the cancer can be detected in the same way.

Still another test is for HCG, human chorionic gonadotropin. HCG is normally present during pregnancy, and serves as a test for that condition. However, if found in a male or a nonpregnant female, HCG is sure evidence of tumors in the uterus, testicles, or even the lungs. This test can be used to detect very early signs of tumor recurrence in those areas.

As with HCG, the unexpected production of various hormones by tumors in other parts of the body can lead to their detection. Medullary carcinoma of the thyroid gland releases calcitonin, which is measurable in the blood by radioimmunoassay. Lung tumors are often capable of secreting such diverse hormones as ADH, antidiuretic hormone; ACTH, adrenocorticotropic hormone; or a substance similar to PTH, parathyroid hormone. In addition, tumors of the endocrine glands often secrete the typical hormone products of those glands.

These various cancer tests, which are either being put into ever-broadening use or are still in the formative stage, are a promising start. Whether it will happen in a decade or a quarter-century, testing for a wide array of cancers by means of a blood or urine sample is bound to become routine.

## Testing for Allergies

There is probably not an allergy sufferer who is not familiar with the traditional skin scratch test. By breaking the surface of the skin and exposing body tissues to minute amounts of the suspected substance, the physician is able to gauge the degree of allergy. For every suspected substance, there is the discomfort of a scratch—and the possibility of an unpleasant reaction if the response is strongly positive.

The new radioallergosorbent test, RAST, which is gaining increasing acceptance among allergists, does away with the tedious and unpleasant scratch test. With a single small specimen of blood, the laboratory can do all the reactive testing. Many common substances can now be tested by this technique as potential allergens—house dust, weeds, pollens, grasses, animal hairs, foods, or what-have-you.

Allergy testing through the new RAST method may become an increasingly important diagnostic tool in many conditions that do not at first glance appear to be allergy-related. Allergies can cause not only such familiar symptoms as a rash or a runny nose, but virtually any symptom described in this book, from headaches to coma or death. By eliminating the scratch test, availability of the simple RAST may prompt even non-allergists to order such a test in some hard-to-diagnose conditions.

The cost of RAST is still substantial, and the number of suspected allergens for which the test can be used is still relatively limited. As this number expands—and as further automation brings down the cost—RAST testing may someday become a part of a complete physical examination.

## Chemical Messengers and Prostaglandins

Already able to detect infinitesimal changes in blood, urine, and other bodily specimens, laboratory testing is likely to become still further refined. Scientists are working on understanding the complex system of chemical communication that goes on continuously within each cell. It is a most subtle process, with sending and receiving units conveying chemical messages between different parts of the cell.

What researchers have found is that if this delicate process of communication within each cell is somehow disrupted, clinical diseases occur. Many new diagnostic methods will be developed from these studies. In some cases, a chemical messenger can be sent into the cells. If it returns to the bloodstream properly modified, the system is working. But if it returns unchanged, or incorrectly changed, there is a defect in that system.

A remarkable example of putting this method to use is in resolving the problem of ambiguous genitalia in the newborn. This condition, in which the baby's genitals have an appearance midway between the sexes, is sometimes caused by a deficiency of a special enzyme called 5-alpha-reductase. Under normal circumstances, this enzyme converts the male hormone, testosterone, to a much more powerful derivative, dihydrotestosterone. By giving an injection of testosterone and measuring the appearance of its expected product in the bloodstream, a deficiency of the enzyme can be detected, and the proper sex identification made. Hormone treatments and appropriate surgical corrections can then help the baby assume its proper sex. Many potential physical and emotional problems in the years to come can thus be headed off.

Another type of blood analysis that will increase in scope is the "search and identify" type of chemical messenger. A substance known as technetium isotope, for example, can find its way to tumor cells and areas of arthritis, whereupon it broadcasts a cluster of radiation. Scanning electronic equipment will then identify the site. There is a new test for damaged heart muscle based on accumulation of thallium isotope. Another test using gallium isotope can reveal pockets of infection deep in the abdominal organs. Radioactive cholesterol can search out and identify very small adrenal tumors.

These are but a few of many similar tests that are on the drawing boards. In a sense, these tests bring the test to the tissue rather than bring the tissue to the laboratory. We can expect many more ideas and inventions in this field.

Prostaglandins are another class of substances in your body which may offer exciting opportunities for diagnosis through laboratory testing. Known since the 1930s, prostaglandins are presently being investigated with the purpose of explaining some of the body's cellular reactions to various diseases and abnormal conditions.

Prostaglandins may possibly be the individual cell's messenger system for informing the body how to react. Acting together with the body's hormones, they control cell activity at the minutest level.

Prostaglandins are made from the fatlike substances in the cell membranes of most tissues. From the instant of their formation, they have an immediate and direct effect on the body. Fever, shock, bronchial asthma, diarrhea, hypertension, allergies, and tissue inflammation may all be in part provoked by the formation of certain prostaglandin substances.

Aspirin and similar compounds inhibit the formation of prostaglandins, thus providing one explanation of the role of aspirin in reducing inflammation. Insufficient prostaglandins may be indirectly involved in constipation, peptic ulcers, and possibly even male sterility—since sperm has increased motility when certain prostaglandins are present.

Prostaglandins are also receiving attention for use as contraceptive agents. When minute amounts are added to the vaginal canal, the womb contracts, preventing the implantation of a fertilized egg.

Medical science is just beginning to learn about prostaglandins and their effects on the body. As knowledge of these chemicals expands and laboratory testing capabilities are refined, then controlling the quantity and use of the body's prostaglandin system may be a tool for the future physician to treat disorders which are difficult to manage today.

## New Technology

Among the most notable advances of the past several years is the continual reduction in the time it takes to obtain the results for some of the most basic blood tests. Not only the autoanalyzer, which can turn out as many as twenty-four different kinds of tests on literally thousands of samples, but other, comparable devices with space-age response capability are now standard laboratory equipment.

But such advances do not always require complex machinery. We take for granted, for example, the "dipstick" analysis of a urine sample for six or more substances. How convenient it would be if the physician could perform a similar test on a sample of blood in the office. In due time, this too should be possible.

One dramatic advance that is almost ready now is a direct analysis by a tiny probe inserted within a blood vessel. The probe sends out continuous readings. Among the blood constituents which probes are now capable of analyzing are blood sugar, carbon dioxide, salt concentrations, calcium, and pH. Probes that could be made sensitive to many other chemicals in the bloodstream are on the drawing boards. New principles, such as nuclear magnetic resonance, or NMR, are being used to detect even minor differences between complex molecules.

Considerable development can be expected in the amount of information medical laboratories will be able to provide to doctors. This could be in the form of a central computerized system with remote terminals and telephone access lines right in the doctor's office. Doctors would thus have immediate access to the most detailed, up-to-date information that may be relevant to specific test results of individual patients.

For example, the physician has just received the results of a certain combination of liver-function tests. Noting possible inconsistencies between the test results and the actual physical examination of the patient, the doctor has some questions. What diseases are possible with this group of results? What medications give false positive results? How many weeks after onset of hepatitis will test results remain above normal levels? What percentage of a normal population sample could have those results and remain free of known disease? What are the norms for a woman in the second trimester of pregnancy? Instantly, those answers will flash on a display screen or be automatically typed out, to become part of the patient's permanent medical record.

Astounding as some of the advances of coming years may turn out to be, no one should expect that everything he or she hears about in the various media will come true. Hardly a week goes by without a major story of some exciting new discovery or breakthrough in the field of medical laboratory testing. Whatever the discovery or breakthrough, it will usually take years to check it out, and then years more to give it a practical application on a routine basis. Along the way, many of these unconfirmed discoveries will be greatly modified or discarded altogether.

Others, however, will eventually come to fruition. Considering the tremendous amount of activity in this field, even a relatively low rate of success will result in spectacular progress.

To speculate on all the future possibilities of medical laboratory testing is an interesting exercise. What is more important is that we fully utilize the laboratory tests at our disposal today, so that we may enjoy the best possible health—today and tomorrow.

# Appendix.
# At a Glance:
# Additional Common Tests

*Adrenocorticotropic Hormone (ACTH)*

ACTH is a hormone released by the pituitary gland to stimulate the adrenal glands to produce and release primarily cortisol. Certain cancerous tumors in varying parts of the body may release ACTH as a by-product of the malignancy process.

*Aldolase*

This chemical is an enzyme which helps metabolize fructose. Fructose is a sugar found in muscles, and its abnormal presence in serum is usually associated with muscle disease. Elevated aldolase levels may be found with heart and liver damage and in certain cancers and anemias.

*Amylase*

Amylase is a group of enzymes produced in the pancreas, salivary glands, liver, and Fallopian tubes. The function of amylase is to break down starch into smaller sugar units which are further digested to glucose. This enzyme usually is analyzed to determine the possibility of an irritated or inflamed pancreas. Significantly increased serum levels of amylase are found with disorders of the pancreas or with intestinal obstructions.

*Antinuclear Antibody (ANA)*

Systemic lupus erythematosus (SLE) causes the body to produce an abnormal class of unique antibodies which can be detected with the antinuclear antibody procedure. Special fluoresein-labeled antiserum is used to identify the ANA with the aid of a fluorescent-light-field microscope. In addition to lupus, other conditions which can yield a positive result include rheumatoid arthritis, colitis, hepatitis, and infectious mononucleosis.

### Antistreptolysin Titer (ASOT)

Infections by the microorganisms in the Group A streptococcal family cause the body to produce anti-streptococcal antibodies. Youngsters between the ages of five and thirteen are continually exposed to these organisms and sometimes have symptoms of a "strep throat" infection. Measuring the level of ASOT is used to determine the presence of the infection and the progress of recovery.

### Carcinoembryonic Antigen (CEA)

This antigen is a protein usually associated with certain cancers of the lungs, breasts, colon, and prostate gland. The amount of antigen found in healthy non-smoking individuals is less than 2 nanograms per milliliter. In excess of 5 nanograms, the antigen may signify the development of an unsuspected cancer, or the elevation could be caused by cirrhosis, ulcers, colitis, or heavy smoking. CEA tests are also performed after cancer surgery to assess the possibility of any cancerous tissues remaining.

### Catecholamines

Catecholamines are a general class of chemicals produced in the central core of the adrenal glands. These chemicals are epinephrine and norepinephrine, both used by the body to respond quickly to stressful stimulation. Epinephrine causes the heart to increase its pulse rate and activates the breakdown of stored glucose into a form for quick energy. Norepinephrine increases both diastolic and systolic blood pressure. Catecholamines help prepare the individual for "fight or flight" in stressful situations. The analysis of catecholamines in a twenty-four-hour urine specimen is used to determine potential problems with the medullary portion of the adrenal gland, particularly when high blood pressure is evident. Elevations of catecholamines can signify the presence of an adrenal tumor such as a pheochromocytoma in adults and neuroblastoma in children.

### C-Reactive Protein (CRP)

CRP is a protein which is detectable in various infections and inflammatory conditions. The determination of CRP can be used to monitor the progress of recuperation from these inflammatory problems. The CRP test is more sensitive than the ESR, erythrocyte sedimentation rate, and is not as unstable after a time delay in analyzing the blood. CRP is often used to monitor patients with rheumatoid arthritis or with fever.

### Delta Amino Levulinic Acid

This organic acid is an intermediary product in the synthesis of the heme portion of hemoglobin. Its abnormal presence in urine indicates an interruption in the synthesis of heme found in hemoglobin, observed in intermittent porphyria and in lead poisoning. It may also be elevated in certain liver disorders.

### Electrophoresis: Lipoproteins

This procedure is used to separate, under the influence of an electrical gradient, the cholesterol-containing proteins of serum. The following classes of lipid-containing proteins are separated: alpha, beta, and pre-beta lipoproteins and chylomicrons, which are primarily triglycerides.

### Electrophoresis: Proteins

This procedure is used to separate, under the influence of an electrical field, the various protein constituents of serum in order to determine their relative concentration. The following protein groups are identifiable: albumin, alpha globulins, beta globulins, and gamma globulins.

### 5-prime-Nucleotidase

This enzyme is found in the liver. Its measurement in serum is used to differentiate obstructive jaundice or lesions of the liver from bone cell disorders. If the patient is jaundiced because of elevated bilirubin or if the patient has an elevated alkaline phosphatase result, the 5-prime-nucleotidase test may be ordered to identify the specific disorder.

### Glycohemoglobin

Persistent high levels of glucose in the blood combine to some extent with the hemoglobin of red blood cells. This combination can be measured as glycohemoglobin, which is related to the amount of glucose elevation and the duration of exposure to it. This test is used to monitor the relative blood sugar level during the three months prior to the test and is useful to the physician in determining the severity of diabetes mellitus and the individual patient's compliance with the treatment program.

## Hepatitis Associated Antigen (HAA)

This test is used to detect and confirm the presence of hepatitis infection. The serum is usually analyzed by the techniques of radioimmunoassay. A positive confirmation may not be made until the virus has incubated and then reproduced itself in the liver. This could take from few weeks to a few months after the initial exposure to the hepatitis-causing virus.

## Isocitric Dehydrogenase

This enzyme is found mainly in the liver, and as with SGPT, an elevation is indicative of some form of liver damage. Significantly high levels are found in viral hepatitis infection. Lower levels are found in cirrhosis and obstructive jaundice.

## Lipase

Lipase is an enzyme which digests triglycerides into their subunits. The enzyme is produced mainly in the pancreas. As with amylase, the elevation of lipase in serum is associated with inflammation and other disorders of the pancreas.

## Metanephrines

Metanephrines are the breakdown products of catecholamines, epinephrine and norepinephrine. The amount of metanephrines found in a twenty-four-hour urine specimen is greater than for catecholamines, but usually less than for VMA. Because of the chemical breakdown pathways used during the presence of tumors, some patients who have a pheochromocytoma may have normal catecholamines but increased metanephrines.

## Mono Spot/Heterophile

The presence of mononucleosis is determined by analyzing a few drops of blood with the sensitive mono spot test. If the result is positive, then the extent of infection is determined by making dilutions of the blood serum and assaying the diluted serum utilizing the antibodies contained in the heterophile procedure. When an individual complains of stomach pains, swollen glands, sore throat, and headache, the mono spot test may be performed to rule out—or confirm—infectious mononucleosis.

## Osmolality

Osmolality is a test to measure the osmotic pressure of blood or urine resulting from the amount of various salts and other chemicals present. This test is somewhat more accurate than the specific gravity test discussed in the urinalysis section. It is usually performed when salt imbalance, kidney damage, uncontrolled diabetes, or any degree of excess water loss or retention is suspected.

## Rheumatoid Factor

Antibodies associated with rheumatoid arthritis can be detected through serological techniques. The body often produces antibodies against its own injured tissues, and the presence of such a finding is associated with many diseases. In addition to rheumatoid arthritis, these include such inflammatory conditions as bronchitis, asthma, asbestosis, hepatitis, and cirrhosis.

## 17-Hydroxycorticosteroids

This chemical test is performed on a twenty-four-hour collection of urine and measures the mixture of substances formed from cortisol, a major product of the adrenal glands. The results indicate the daily secretion of the adrenal glands and are used to assess under or overactivity of the pituitary-adrenal glandular system. Above normal values are found with excess secretion of pituitary ACTH (see page 113), adrenal gland tumor, or stress states. Obesity or certain tranquilizer drugs may falsely elevate the result. Below normal values are observed in Addison's disease or deficiency of pituitary ACTH. Decreased levels may also be caused by hypothyroidism, liver disease, prolonged bed rest, anorexia nervosa or advanced age. A simultaneous measurement of creatinine is used to correct the result for individual differences in body weight and kidney function.

## 17-Ketosteroids

This group of substances is measured in a twenty-four-hour collection of urine and represents the products derived from male hormones secreted primarily by the adrenal glands and, to a lesser extent, by the testes or ovaries. The values are higher in males compared to females, and higher in the teen- to mid-twenty age group. Lowest values are observed before puberty and after the menopause. Increased amounts of 17-Ketosteroids can be caused by excessive secretion of pituitary or tumor ACTH, adrenal gland tumors, cancer of the adrenal glands, rare testicular tumors, or hereditary disorders of adrenal gland hormone production known as the adrenogenital syndrome. Decreased levels are observed with inadequate pituitary ACTH function or Addison's disease of the adrenal glands. As with 17-hydroxycorticosteroids, certain tranquilizer drugs may cause falsely elevated values. Likewise, measurement of creatinine is used to adjust the results for differences in body weight and kidney function.

## Vanillylmandelic Acid (VMA)

This chemical is the end product of catecholamine breakdown, whereas metanephrine is the precursor chemical to VMA. VMA is found normally in a twenty-four-hour urine specimen in greater concentrations than for catecholamines and metanephrines. Its elevation usually signifies the increased production and excretion of catecholamines by a tumor of the adrenal glands, or of the chromaffin system, made up of sympathetic nerve nodes which lie within the abdomen and deep within the chest cavity.

# Index